DEALING WITH QUESTIONS ABOUT SEX

by Arlene Uslander and Caroline Weiss
with the editors of LEARNING magazine

AF717704

PLEASE RETURN TO LIBRARY
PLANNED PARENTHOOD: SHASTA-DIABLO
2185 PACHECO STREET
CONCORD, CA 94520
(510) 676-0505

LEARNING Handbooks
530 University Avenue
Palo Alto, California 94301

FOREWORD

Questions, misunderstandings and apprehensions about sex *can* be handled in a relaxed, non-threatening way. This handbook describes a humanistic approach which lets children learn through discussion—*when* they are ready for it. Practical suggestions help you to cope with misconceptions and anxieties; specific answers to questions children ask are also included.

The purpose of this and other LEARNING Handbooks is to help make teaching and learning more effective, interesting and exciting. Arlene Uslander and Caroline Weiss have been involved in teaching sex education for nine years. Their extensive experience has been combined with LEARNING magazine's research facilities and editorial depth to produce this down-to-earth and lively handbook.

Editor: Carol B. Whiteley
Illustrations: By elementary grade children responding to key issues raised in the text
Photography: Ed Lettau
Cover: Illustration by Robert Ryder and Michael Shenon

Executive Editor: Morton Malkofsky
Design Director: Robert G. Bryant

Copyright © 1975, Education Today Company, Inc., 530 University Avenue, Palo Alto, California 94301. World Rights Reserved. No part of this publication may be reproduced by any mechanical, photographic, or electronic process, or in any other form, nor may it be stored in a retrieval system, transmitted, or otherwise copied for public or private use without prior written permission from Education Today Company, Inc.

Library of Congress Number: 75-12460
International Standard Book Number: 0-915092-04-2

Book Code: 007 • Second Printing July 1977

CONTENTS

1 SEX EDUCATION AND THE SCHOOL 4

2 PREPARING CLASS, SCHOOL AND COMMUNITY 10

3 PREPARING YOURSELF 18

4 GETTING STARTED 26

5 HOLDING DISCUSSIONS 34

6 TALKING TO CHILDREN ABOUT SEX 46

7 TALKING ABOUT GROWING UP 60

8 QUESTIONS AND ANSWERS 68

9 GLOSSARY 80

10 RESOURCES 90

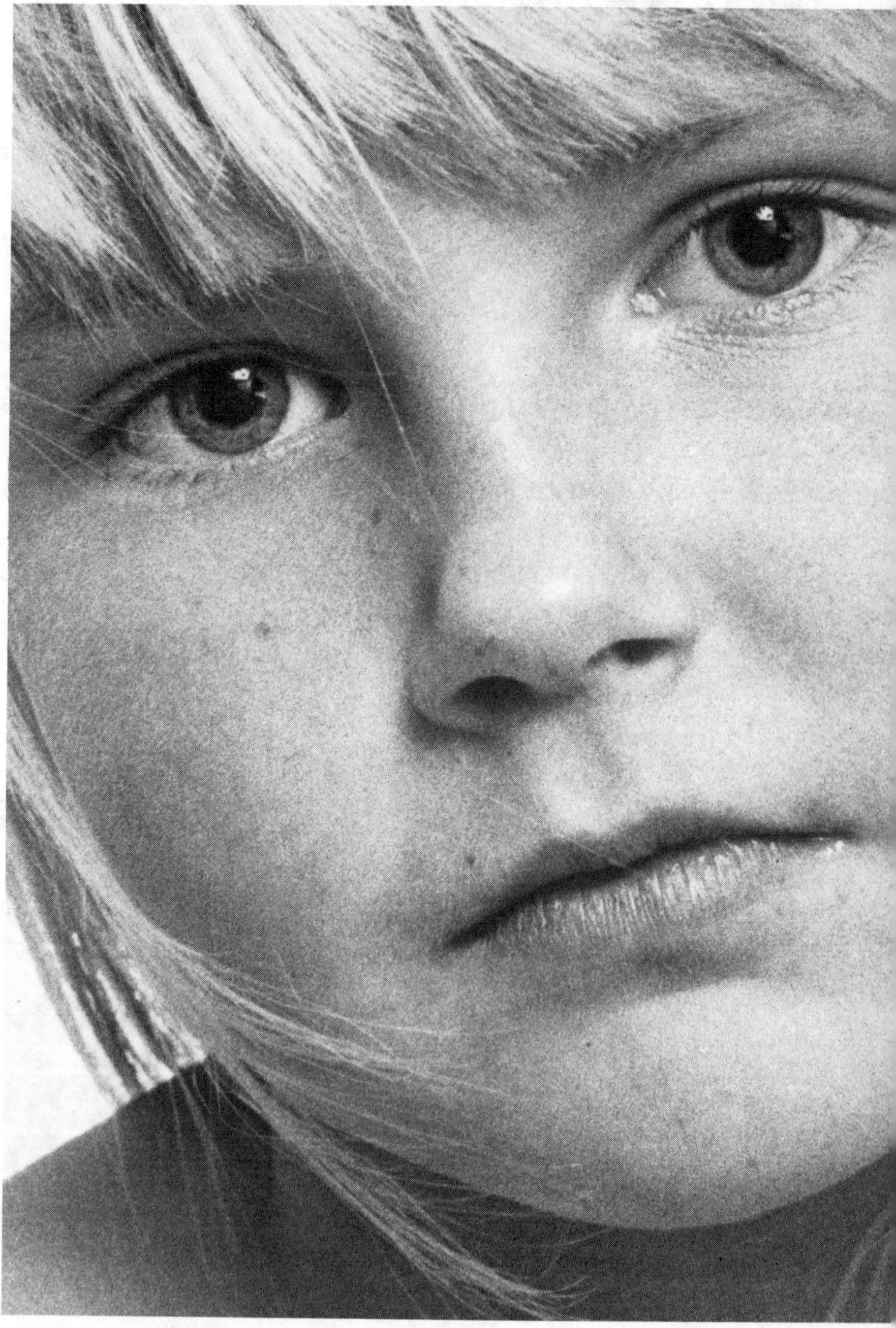

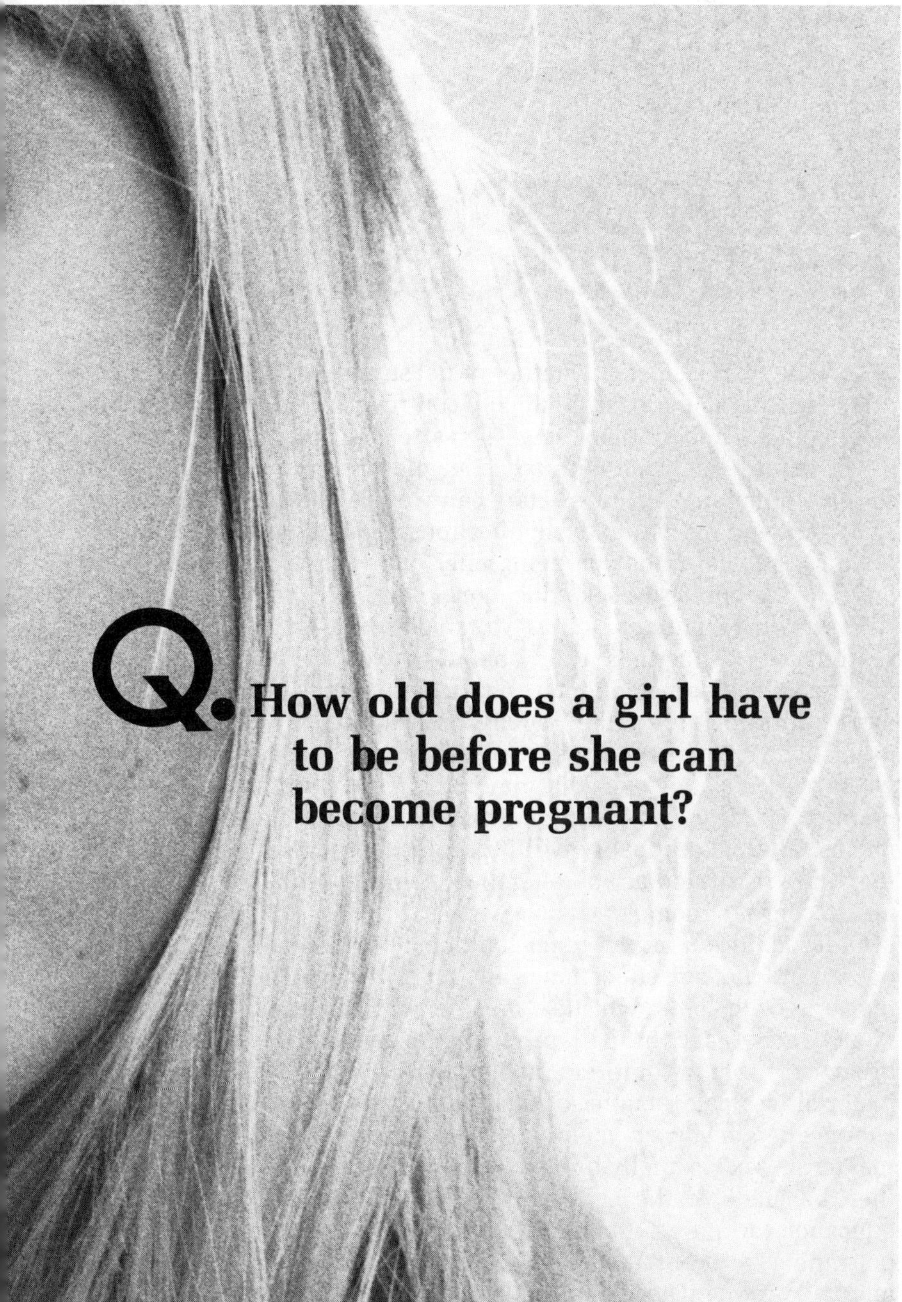

Q. How old does a girl have to be before she can become pregnant?

CHAPTER 1

SEX EDUCATION AND THE SCHOOL

THE QUESTION of whether or not sex education belongs in the school is no longer the highly controversial issue it was at one time. The question now seems to be, how can our schools provide children with sex education programs which are not simply "plumbing" courses? How can we provide children with the opportunity to discuss and ask questions about all aspects of human behavior, sexual behavior being only one aspect? In other words, how can we *humanize* sex education?

There are a number of things we can do. To begin with, we can give sex education programs a new name — we can replace the easily misunderstood and emotionally charged term "sex education" with a more appropriate name, such as "Human Relations," "Life Education" or "The Study of People." There are several reasons why we suggest this. For one, you may have a difficult time trying to explain to younger children what the term "sex education" actually means. The kids probably will be confused and you, no doubt, will feel quite frustrated as you attempt to come up with a definition that makes sense to them.

Older children, on the other hand, may have many preconceived notions of what sex education is all about — they're apt to respond to the term with leers, whistles, laughter or considerable embarrassment. Such reactions will probably be avoided if the subject is broached from a different angle. By discussing sexually tinged material in a calm, matter-of-fact manner, under a less emotionally charged heading, we can eliminate the stigma or myth before the actual term "sex" is finally brought into the conversation. The point can then be made to the children that they have been receiving sex education for quite a while and weren't even aware of it; this should help them to understand that sex education consists of more than merely learning where babies come from. At this point, the children may want to name or rename their program themselves.

Still another reason for choosing a different name for the program is that many parents feel extremely apprehensive about their children learning sexual information in school — they, too, have preconceived notions of what sex education consists of. If they can be assured that their children are involved in a program in which the discussion of feelings is just as important as the imparting of facts, they will probably feel much less threatened and your job will be an easier one. The parent who bristles with anger when his child tells him that he went to his "sex education class" may very well nod his head in complete approval upon hearing that the child participated in something called "Human Relations" or "Sharing with Others."

WHAT SEX EDUCATION REALLY IS

A second step toward humanizing sex education is to decide what it really is — what it really should be. One way to determine this is to decide what it is not — what we don't want it to be. Sex education should not be merely the imparting of physiological facts of reproduction or venereal disease. It should not merely give information on the mechanics of birth control. Nor should it be a two-week unit or once a year crash course on the human body, designed to meet the requirements of a science curriculum.

Sex education in our schools should be a whole communication process between adult and child and between child and child; it should be based upon openness, honesty and mutual respect. Sex education has to do with feelings and people and relationships, but it becomes meaningful to children only when it relates to their own needs, their own concerns, their own fears. A sex education program should encourage each child to discuss anything that is of interest, importance or concern to him, regardless of whether it is the loss of a baby tooth or the loss of an unborn baby in the family.

Because it deals with feelings and relationships, sex education can help children become more sensitive to the needs of others; it can help them to understand how their words and actions affect the feelings and behavior of those around them. Ideally, sex education is a sharing process through which children learn to have an appreciation and respect for the differences between them, and through which they become more conscious of the similarities. "[It] is the imparting of correct physiological information to children, while at the same time trying to instill within them an awareness and acceptance of their own sexuality and of their roles as males or females, and more importantly, as human beings, within the framework of the family, the peer group, and in society."[1]

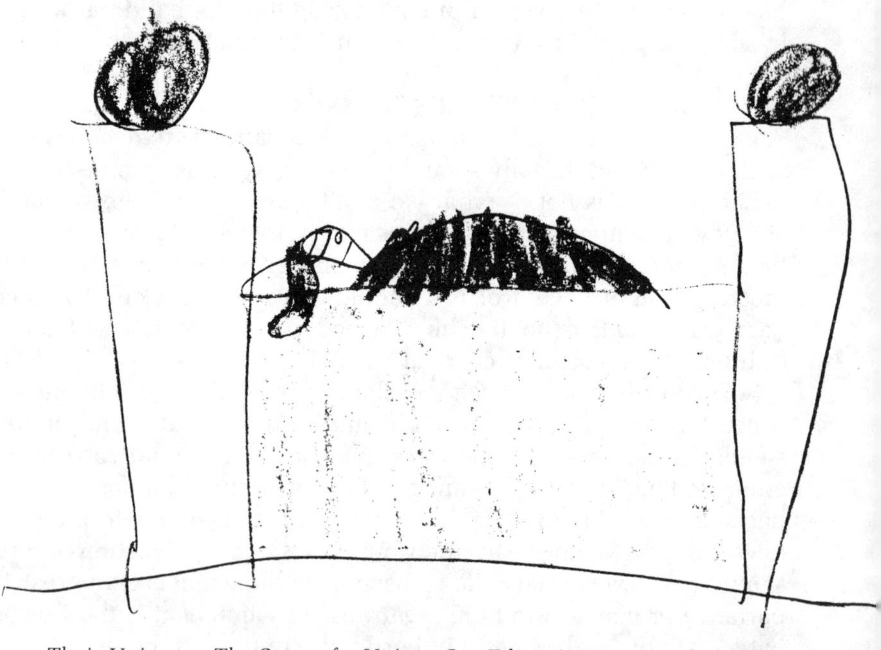

[1]From *Their Universe: The Story of a Unique Sex Education Program for Kids* by Arlene Uslander et al. (New York: Delacorte Press, 1973), p. 146.

Having decided what sex education should be, how do we make it a reality? One school district in a Chicago suburb formulated a program which it felt taught sex education in a humanized, effective way; the program, begun in 1966 and still in operation today, differs from traditional programs in that there is no formal curriculum and no books, films, filmstrips or any other kinds of audio-visual aids. It is a program based on discussion and allows children to talk about anything that is important to them. No grades are given and no specific amount of information is expected to be covered. We have been affiliated with that program since its inception. What follows is a complete description of it — you can modify it as you see fit, to suit the requirements of your students, your school and your community.

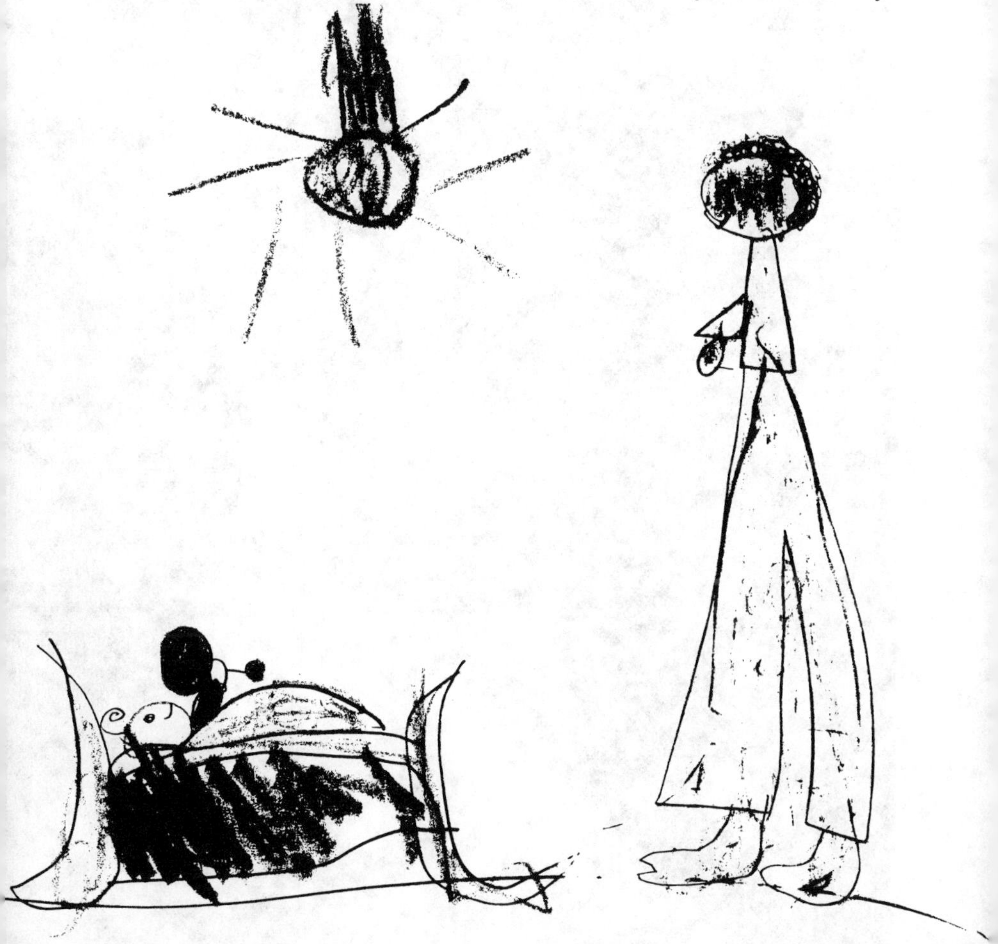

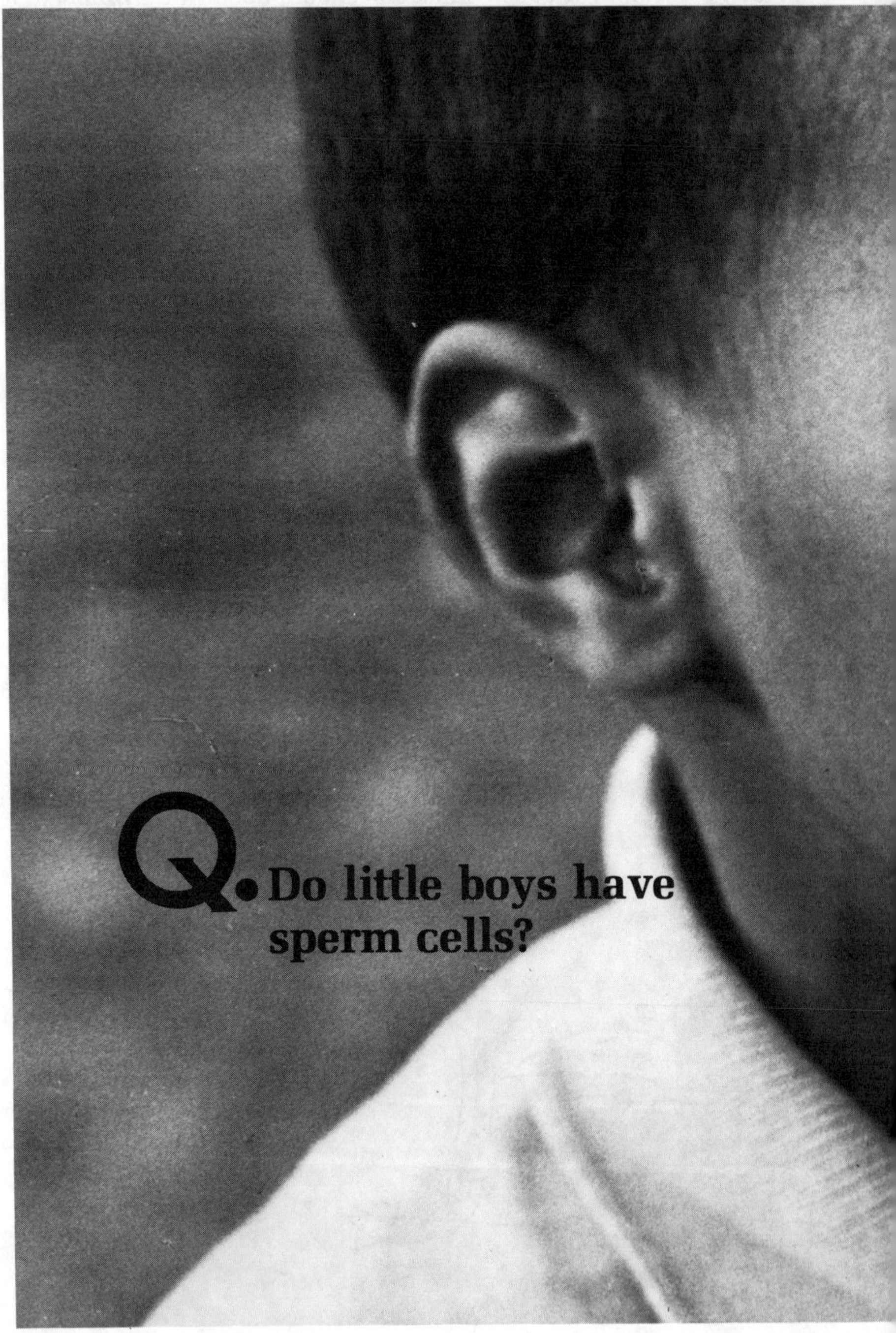
Q. Do little boys have sperm cells?

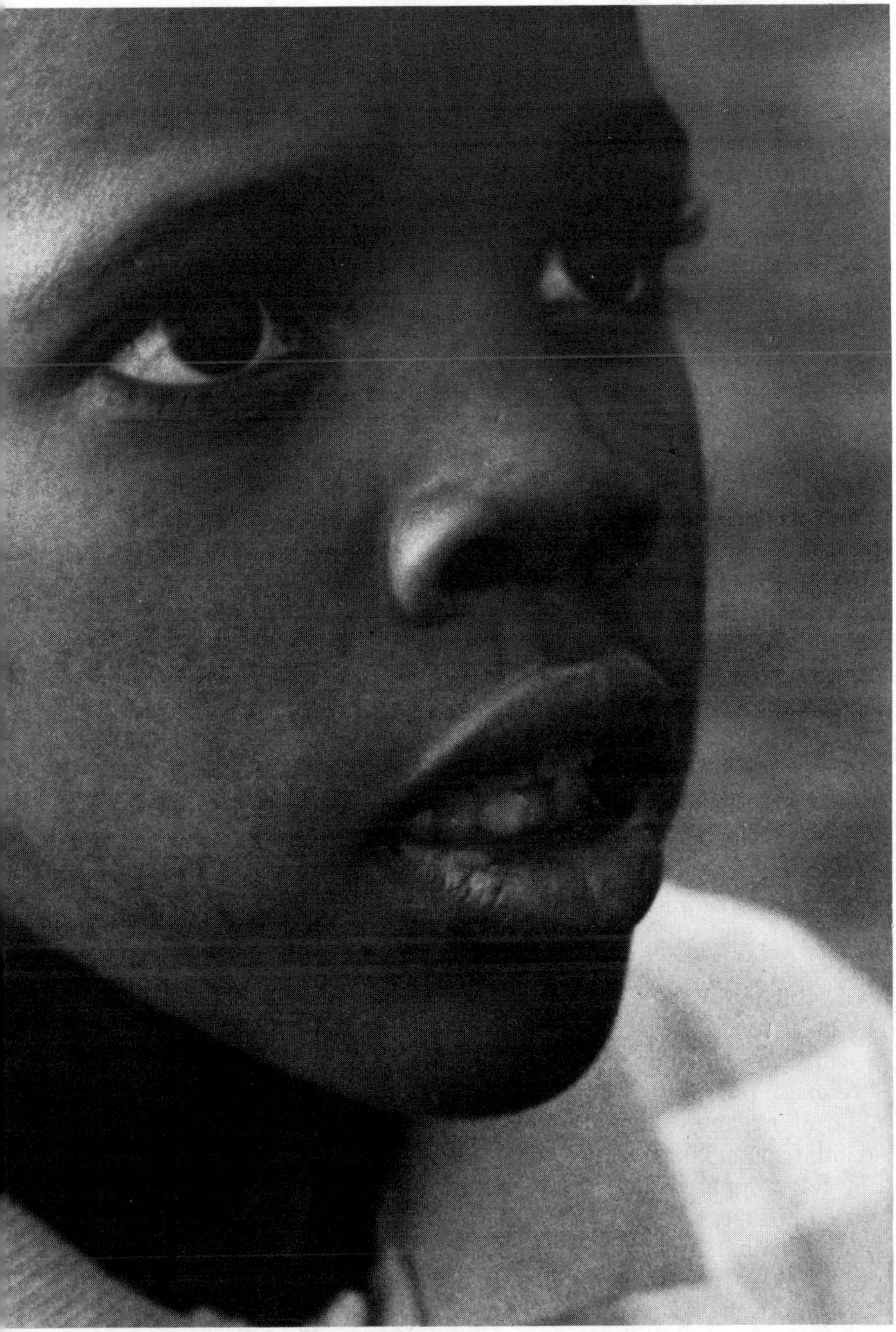

CHAPTER 2

PREPARING CLASS, SCHOOL AND COMMUNITY

BEFORE YOU BEGIN to plan your program, a word of caution — without the cooperation of the parents whose children will be involved, your program will never get off the ground. Strained relationships between parents and administrators may result if parents are unsure or fearful of the project; this tension will undoubtedly be reflected in the attitude of the children, caught in the middle. The fact that parents have the legal right to exclude or withdraw their children from sex education classes makes it doubly important for the school district to have parental approval.

We suggest that meetings between parents, teachers and school administrators be held during the planning stages of this addition to the traditional curriculum; continue the meetings on a regular basis after the program has begun. Parents should be fully informed about the nature of thc program, its costs and the kinds of people who will be working with their children. They will need constant reassurance until they are satisfied that the school is not usurping their role as parents, but merely supplementing that role by assisting both parent and child to communicate with one another and with society. Continued parental support will insure your program's success.

A GENERAL DESCRIPTION OF THE PROGRAM

The basic format of our sex education program is one of open-ended conversation between small groups of children and an adult leader. A relaxed and comfortable atmosphere allows discussion of sexual material in a natural way, simulating as closely as possible the kind of sexual discussions parents would have with their children at home if they felt competent and comfortable in doing so. The program permits children to talk about anything that is of interest, importance and concern to them, and provides correct sexual information when and if the topic is introduced by the children themselves. It is a program that *allows* sex education to happen, rather than *forcing* it to happen.

Each child (within his or her own group) is given an opportunity to speak — often, whatever the child is interested in at that particular moment becomes the subject of discussion for that day. This means that there can be a number of different subjects mentioned during a meeting, or only one subject, if it holds the interest and attention of the group for the entire time. In the first few weeks there may be only "small talk," centering around vacations, pets, television programs, etc. But those weeks of seemingly unimportant chatter will be well spent in establishing a feeling of rapport and trust among the children, and between the children and you.

To those of you who are asking at this point, "But what if the children never bring up the subject of sex?" we would like to point out that in all the years we have been working in the field of sex education, we have *never* had a group of youngsters who didn't bring it up eventually. Just as adults will discuss sex when they feel comfortable with a group of friends, so will children. After an exchange of views and ideas in the group meetings, children will understand that sex is an acceptable topic of conversation, because it is an acceptable part of life.

WHO SHOULD TEACH SEX EDUCATION?

It is the adult discussion leader's role to relax and listen to whatever the children have to say. This means that you must be a flexible, compassionate, non-critical listener. Rather than trying to teach children from your knowledge and experience, you must be open and receptive to children who want to share *their* thoughts and experiences. It may be hard to do this at first, but with time, your role should become more natural.

Not all teachers, however, are capable or want to be sex educators. You may find a colleague who applauds your program but doesn't feel able to introduce it to her class. You may wish to work with her class, too, in exchange for her taking the rest of the classes while you work with one group.

An important part of working with this program is erasing from your mind any preconceived notions that you may have about a child's behavior and ability in the classroom. Regard all the children in a new light — they may respond in a completely different way to this new situation. If you are at all negative, those feelings will be easily transmitted to the children by your tone of voice, facial expressions and gestures. The result can be an awkward, unpleasant — even emotionally damaging — experience for all concerned.

WHEN SHOULD SEX EDUCATION BEGIN?

We recommend that the humanistic approach to sex education be started as early as possible in a child's school career, preferably in kindergarten or first grade. In this way, children will learn as soon as possible to become more sensitive to the needs of others, as well as to their own needs. You can, of course, start the program at any grade level. However, because older children probably will have acquired many inhibitions regarding sex and won't be used to openly discussing their feelings in school, a much longer conditioning period will probably be necessary before the children in the group will feel sufficiently at ease to speak freely and relate to one another.

WHERE SHOULD THE MEETINGS TAKE PLACE?

If possible, the children should leave their regular classroom and meet with you in an informal setting, conducive to relaxed conversation, where they will not be distracted by thoughts or physical reminders of school work. But while a small, private room would be perfect, any space in your classroom with enough room for a circle of chairs will work. Weather permitting, groups can even meet outside.

No matter where you meet, we do not recommend that you seat your groups around a table. After moderating discussions both with and without a table, it is our feeling that a table acts as a barrier to the flow of conversation; groups using a table tend to take longer to establish a relationship than those sitting openly in a circle. Using a table also makes it more difficult to maintain group control and to keep the attention of younger children. Youngsters discover in a very short time that a table conceals a multitude of extraneous activities, such as pinching, poking and toe touching, all of which will prove to be distracting.

GROUP SIZE IS OF GREAT IMPORTANCE

Meet with six to ten children at a time. If a group has fewer members, the children will be under a strain to keep the conversation going. If, on the other hand, the group is too large, children, like adults in a similar situation, will be reluctant to discuss anything of a personal or emotional nature. With six to ten in each group, young children will have an opportunity to speak often and won't become impatient or restless while waiting for a turn. With older children, the small group will promote a feeling of comfort and intimacy, and even the child who is extremely shy should find it easier to speak up.

THE COMPOSITION OF THE GROUPS

Each group should consist of as equal a number of girls and boys as possible. This kind of grouping is important in helping children to understand and respect the physical and emotional differences and samenesses between males and females. It also helps them to feel at ease discussing sexual topics in a mixed group — by the time they reach junior high school or high school where such topics are generally introduced to girls and boys together, they will not experience the acute feelings of discomfort and embarrassment common to most youngsters at that age.

Should a group be selected according to the ability, intelligence or maturity of its members? We think not. Through our experiences, we have found that the most stimulating and exciting discussions occur in those groups that are a combination of all types of children. A group composed solely of the most mature children often lacks spontaneity. These youngsters are apt to hold back, to wait until they are absolutely certain that what they have to say is "the right thing," before they contribute to the conversation. Having learned at a very early age to say what they know adults like to hear, rather than what they themselves really think, it often takes a long time before they dare to be wrong. On the other hand, if the less mature children are grouped together, they tend to be more physical in their behavior — much of the time is spent handling disruptions rather than talking together. By intermingling children in this unique group experience, the more mature youngsters discover that they don't have to be perfect to be accepted, and they in turn have a settling, positive effect upon the less mature members. By selecting your groups at random — alphabetically, counting off numbers or any other method you devise — you will usually arrive at an interesting grouping. If, instead, you decide to group children according to your knowledge of their personalities and abilities, keep in mind that the most interesting discussion groups may be those that group children who at first glance would seem to make the least likely combinations.

Once you have assigned each child to a group, make as few

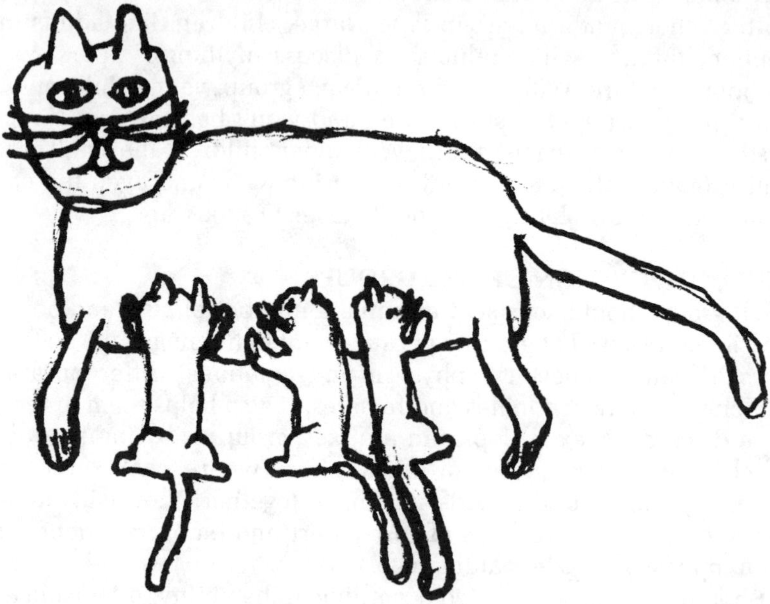

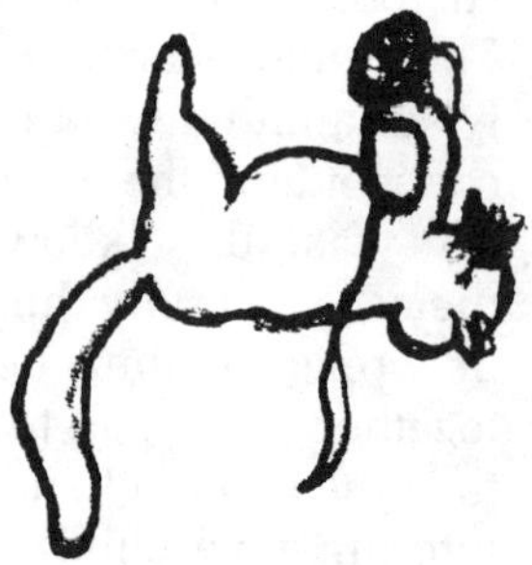

changes as possible during the year. There are some instances, however, when it will be necessary to change one or more children to a different group — a personality clash between certain children may develop or a very uneven mixture of overly talkative and less talkative group members may prove to be detrimental. If, for example, there is one very retiring child within a group of eight or nine outgoing children, it is doubtful that the quiet child will participate very often. Similarly, if most of the members of a group are on the shy side, the one or two talkative youngsters are apt to feel a continuous need to make contributions to the discussion, in order to keep it going.

A conflict in a child's schedule with some other special school program, such as chorus or Student Council, might also necessitate a change. But if it is at all possible, the composition of the groups should remain the same from September until June, so that a feeling of closeness, trust and group belonging can develop.

HOW OFTEN DO THE MEETINGS TAKE PLACE AND HOW LONG DO THEY LAST?

It is our feeling that the group meetings should take place at least once a week and should last for approximately thirty minutes. The half-hour time period is usually adequate, although occasionally you may want to change it. There are times when twenty to twenty-five minutes will be enough for a younger group; other times may find a different group at the same age level frantically waving their hands for additional turns at the end of the thirty minutes. As the children become older, their discussions may get quite involved, possibly extending for forty-five minutes to an hour. But, unless the daily time schedule in your school is unusually flexible, it will be almost impossible to extend the half-hour period on a regular basis.

IS THE PROGRAM WORTH IT?

Generally speaking, the opportunity to discuss fears, concerns and anxieties about life, death, interpersonal relationships and sex is granted only to those children who require the services of a psychiatrist, psychologist or social worker. But what about all the other children who have lesser problems but similar needs?

The humanistic approach to sex education can provide every child in school with an opportunity to talk openly about what they think and feel — are most interested in and worried about — with a listening adult and a group of peers. There is great value in this chance for kids to sit down and talk together, informally, yet on a regular basis. As adults, we derive much comfort and reassurance from hearing a sympathetic friend say to us, "I understand how you feel. I've often felt that way myself." Though a child may use different words — "That's the way it is with me, too," or "That's happened to me" or simply, "Me, too!" — he gets that same feeling of comfort and security from talking openly with his friends.

The sex education program described in this handbook covers far more than merely the physiological "facts of life." It attempts to help children cope with the difficult task of growing up — physically, socially and emotionally. It is education for sharing, and it is education for caring.

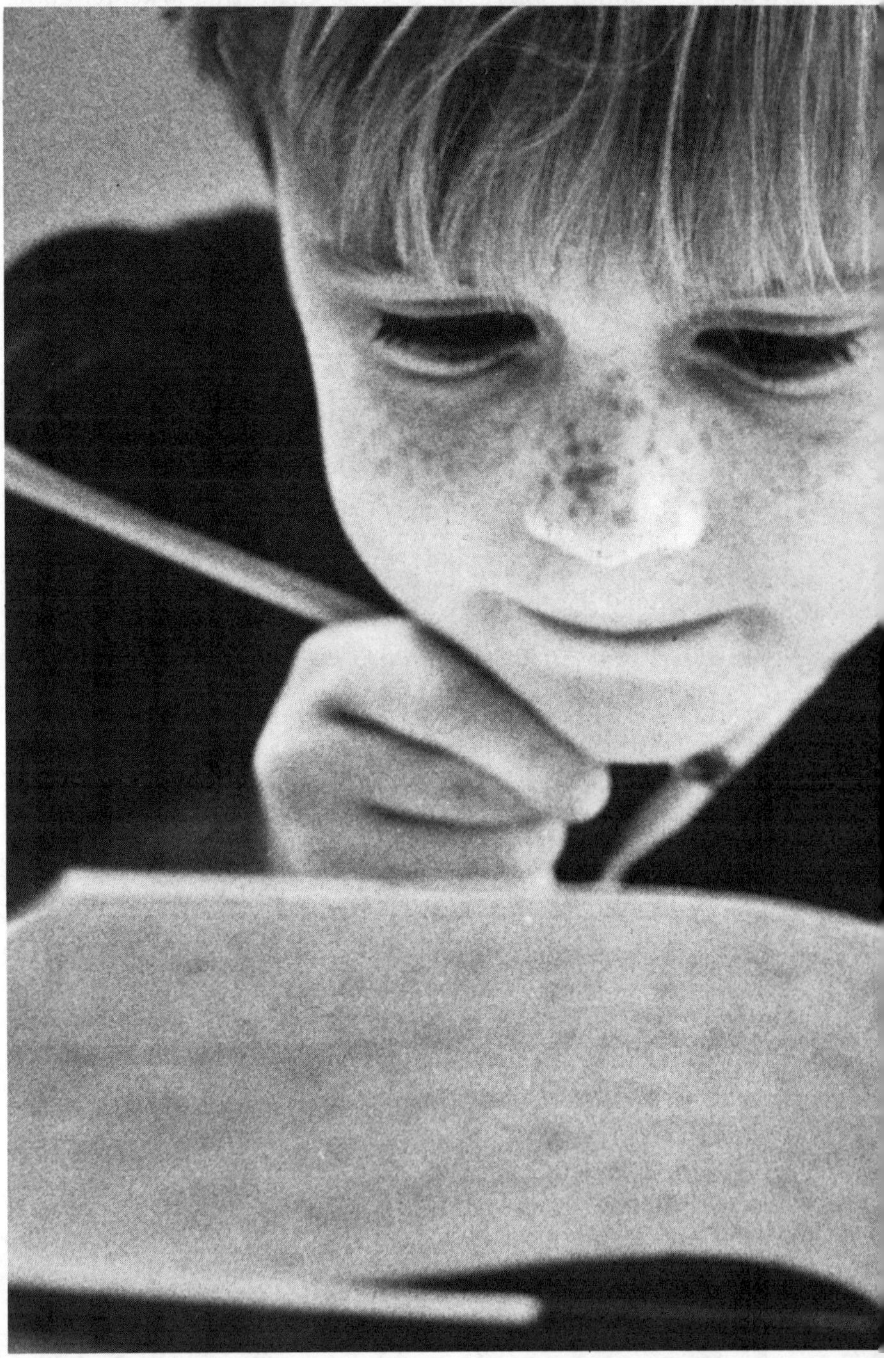

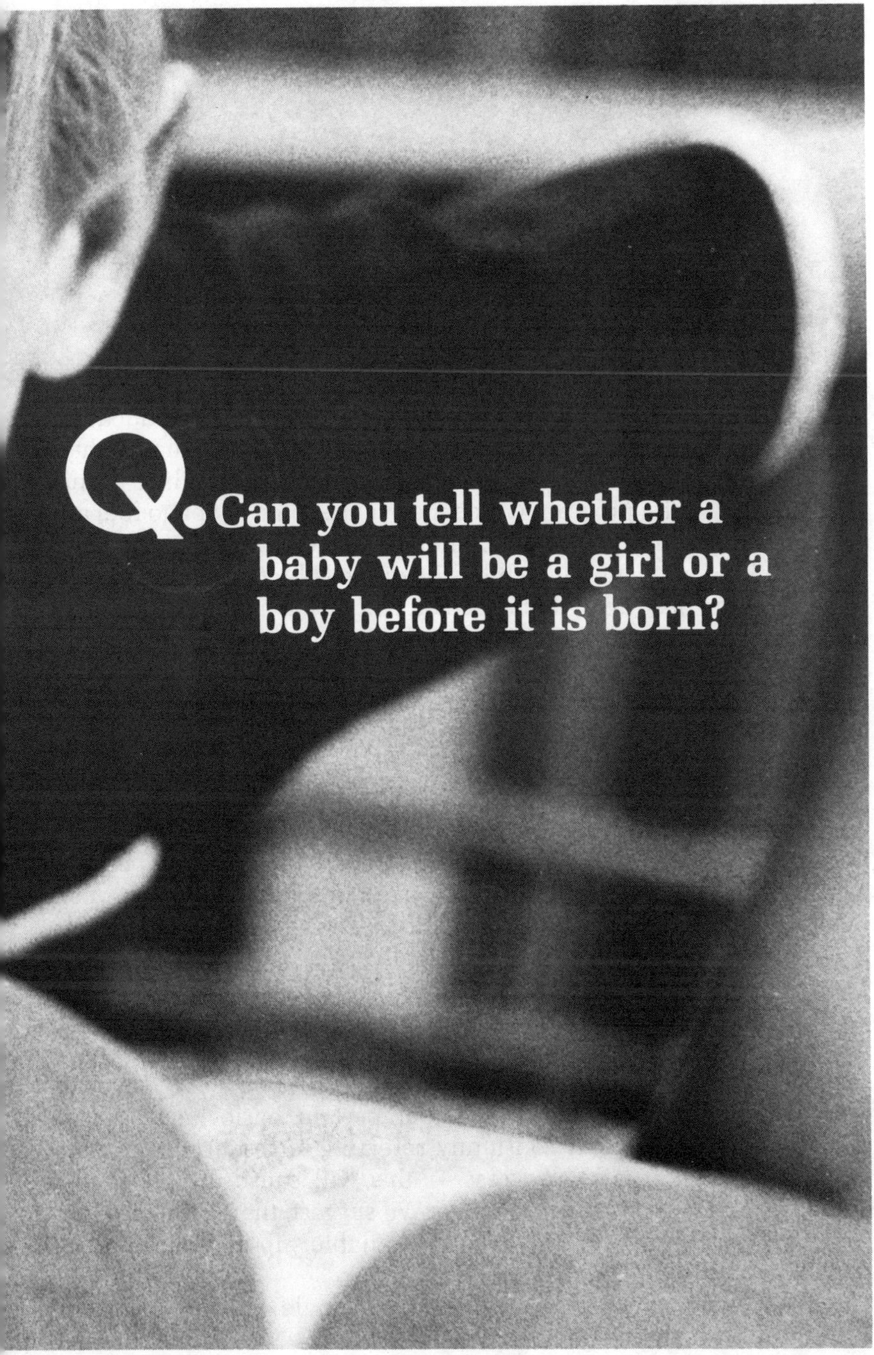

Q. Can you tell whether a baby will be a girl or a boy before it is born?

CHAPTER 3

PREPARING YOURSELF

EVEN THOUGH the humanistic approach to sex education focuses more on feelings than on fact, more on sexuality than on sex, physiological information *will* be covered; it is this aspect of the program which may cause some of you to feel apprehensive. Perhaps you aren't certain that you want to be associated with a field of education which has been the subject of so much controversy in the past, and which necessitates such a high degree of personal involvement. Or perhaps you feel somewhat uncomfortable about discussing topics or using vocabulary which previously haven't been part of your everyday conversations. These are certainly normal reactions!

Once you have been able to overcome your initial reservations, however, you will discover, as we did, that the teaching of sex education can be an extremely rewarding, satisfying and challenging experience. You will realize that few other areas of education provide children with such an excellent opportunity to share feelings. You will realize, furthermore, that few other areas of learning so completely carry over into children's adult lives.

PREPARING TO TEACH SEX EDUCATION

In order to be an effective discussion leader in a program in which sexual topics are spontaneously introduced, you will have to thoroughly understand and remember certain basic facts. If you don't, you'll find yourself constantly referring to resource materials while a discussion is in progress — this will cause the children's enthusiasm and spontaneity to wane. We suggest, therefore, that you read and absorb — beforehand — available, up-to-date material dealing with the following subjects:

1. the physiological development of the male and female from birth through puberty

2. the biological and emotional changes which occur during puberty
3. the story of reproduction and birth for both man and animal

At first glance, this may seem like an overwhelming task. But it isn't necessary for you to spend hour after hour studying complicated technical tomes, acquiring factual knowledge and a vocabulary which, in all probability, you will never need in a teaching situation at the elementary school level. Instead, you can read some of the many excellent, simplified sex-related books and pamphlets written for children; these will supply you with all the correct physiological information and terms you will need to know, and will prepare you to present the information in a way that children can understand.

A list of resource materials which we feel will be particularly helpful to you appears on pages 92–94 of this handbook. We have indicated the books and pamphlets that are most appropriate for each grade level. We would like to point out, however, that adults involved in a sex education program for children should be prepared to discuss a wide range of topics, from the most simple concepts to some that are considerably more advanced. It isn't at all uncommon to hear a six- or seven-year-old ask the kinds of questions we normally expect to hear from much older children. It is also not unusual for a ten-, eleven- or even a twelve-year-old to ask some of the same questions we generally deal with in the primary grades. We strongly recommend, therefore, that you familiarize yourself with the information covered in the resource material suggested for every grade level.

LEARNING FROM THE EXPERIENCES OF OTHERS

Another way to prepare yourself for teaching a sex education program is to seek out colleagues who are currently teaching the subject, and who can share the benefit of their experience with you. We suggest that you arrange to visit on-going sex education classes; seeing for yourself how easily other teachers manage can provide you with a great deal of reassurance.

In-service training, not only in the area of sex education, but, even more importantly, in the area of group dynamics, also would be helpful, though not absolutely necessary. Such training (which should be conducted by a psychologist, a social worker or a guidance counselor who has had considerable experience working with groups of elementary school children) can help prepare you to lead discussion groups and create the informal atmosphere that is necessary to make the program effective.

FEELING AT HOME WITH THE MATERIAL

Many teachers have revealed to us that for them, the most difficult part of teaching sex education — at least in the beginning — was becoming accustomed to calling the reproductive organs by name in the same matter-of-fact manner they discussed any other parts of the body. They felt ill at ease saying such words as "penis," "testicles" and "vagina" in front of a group of children. They also felt uncomfortable using related sex terms, such as "sperm cells," "ova," "menstruation," "sexual intercourse" and the like.

We, too, found it difficult to use the sex education vocabulary when we started out, but we followed some advice given to us by the child psychologist who conducted our training program. We were told to make a list of the words which caused us to feel uncomfortable. We were then advised to say the words over and over again — standing in front of a mirror, driving to work or to the grocery store, conversing with cooperating friends and family. It was also suggested that we repeat the words into a tape recorder and play them back, to get used to hearing our own voices speaking the words aloud. The advice worked — before long, we were able to say the words without feeling embarrassed. More importantly, we were able to help children use the words without feeling embarrassed, and this, of course, is one of the objectives of the program. We discovered that the whole thing was just a matter of conditioning: the more often we said the words, the more comfortable we became using them. You may feel a little foolish saying "penis," "vagina," "uterus" and "breasts" in front of a mirror or into a tape recorder — but the results are well worth it.

The tape recorder also is an invaluable aid that will help you to become a more proficient discussion leader. Hearing your own mistakes on tape can be the most important self-teaching aid available to you. When you use a tape recorder, make sure that the machine is clearly visible and the children know you are taping them and the

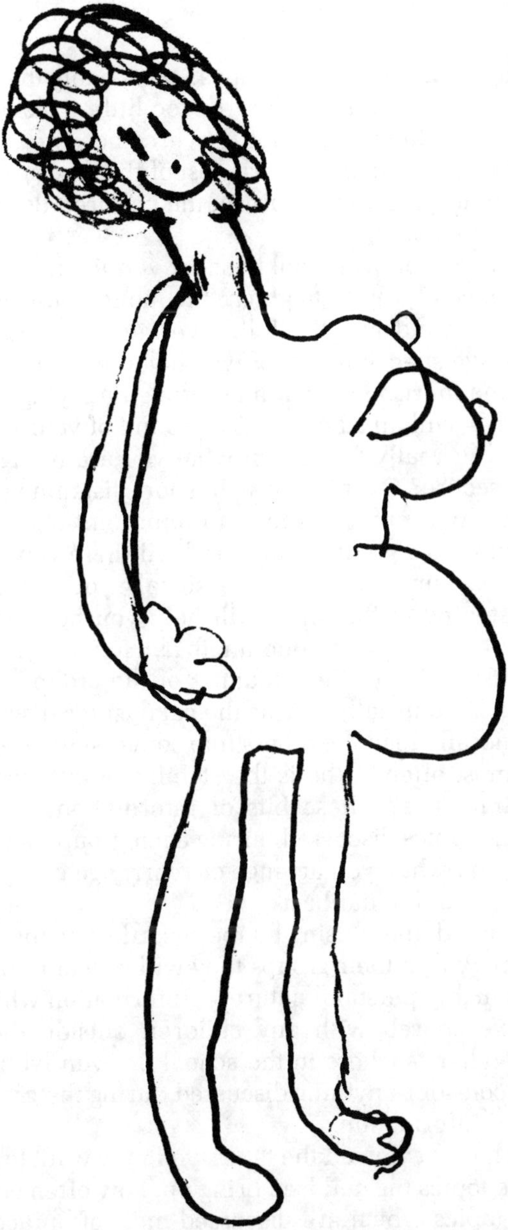

reason for it. The children will probably ask if they can hear themselves on tape. By all means, allow them to. After they have listened to themselves a few times, the novelty will wear off and they will stop asking.

What will you learn from the tapes? Most likely that you have done far too much talking and the children too little. This probably will be one of your most difficult hurdles to overcome, since as a teacher you are no doubt accustomed to doing most of the talking while your class listens. Now, however, you must let the children do most of the talking, while *you* listen.

The tape recorder will frankly show you yourself. You may hear your voice pitched a little too high; the monotone you considered so soothing may sound a trifle dull. Overtalking, pressing to make a point, repetitive speech habits of which you were totally unaware — habits and mannerisms which may prove annoying or disturbing to the children — will all stand out. The sound of your voice will reveal to you how you really feel about what you are doing — a bit tense, perhaps? Insecure? Overanxious? In short, listening to yourself on a tape recorder will provide you with important clues as to how you are functioning as a group leader, and will help you to improve.

Besides becoming aware of the signals you are sending to the children, listening to the tapes will help you become aware of the signals they are sending to one another. Hopefully, you will gain a better understanding of the dynamics of the groups with which you are working: Who usually acts as the catalyst for discussions? Which children generally lead the others into conversations about sex? Who dominates most often? Who is the stabilizing influence? Who is the disturbing influence? These bits of information, along with taped records of the topics discussed during each group meeting, will be of great use to you when you arrange or rearrange groups or work with children on an individual basis.

One final word about using a tape recorder: as the children begin to feel secure within their groups they will reveal information which may be of a highly personal nature — information which they do not want to have shared with any children outside their immediate group, with other teachers in the school or even with their parents. You should consider anything discussed during the group meetings to be privileged information.

After you have reviewed the tapes, you may want to keep a written record of the topics the children bring up, how often each topic is discussed, the topics which are discussed most often according to sex, age level, maturity, etc. These notes can be referred to during future listening sessions.

KEEP WRITTEN RECORDS OF GROUP DISCUSSIONS

Another important aid that will help you to become a more effective discussion leader is to take notes on every session (this can be done as an alternative to taping). It is best to do this as soon as possible after a session is ended, so that what transpired is still fresh in your mind. Write down the different topics that the group talked about. Make a note of any topics that weren't fully discussed because of lack of time, so that you can devote more time to them during another meeting.

If one or more children didn't have sufficient time to talk during a particular session, write down that information. Then you will be sure to call on those children first the next time, if they wish to speak. If a child reveals that he is upset or concerned about something, make a note of that, too, so you will be sure to inquire about how he is feeling the next time you see him.

If you find it difficult to write your notes after a session, you can, if necessary, do it while the discussion is going on. (You may want to do this only if you don't have a tape recorder.) You can learn to take notes unobtrusively, using a clipboard or a small notebook in your lap. These need not be lengthy volumes. By merely jotting down key words or topic headings, you will be able instantly to refresh your memory as to what occurred during a meeting, even after a considerable time lapse. At first, the note taking may be slightly distracting to the children; but if, when they ask, you tell them why you need a written record of the topics covered, they should adjust quickly and soon disregard your scribblings.

BEING A SEX EDUCATOR IS AN ON-GOING PROCESS

Even though we have served as discussion leaders for more than nine years, we still attend sex education workshops, lectures and seminars on group dynamics, read the latest books and re-read some of the older literature in both fields. In addition, we meet on a regular basis with fellow discussion leaders and administrators. Although you will need to acquire the greatest amount of information during the first few months of your new role, training in the areas of group interaction and sex education should be an on-going process.

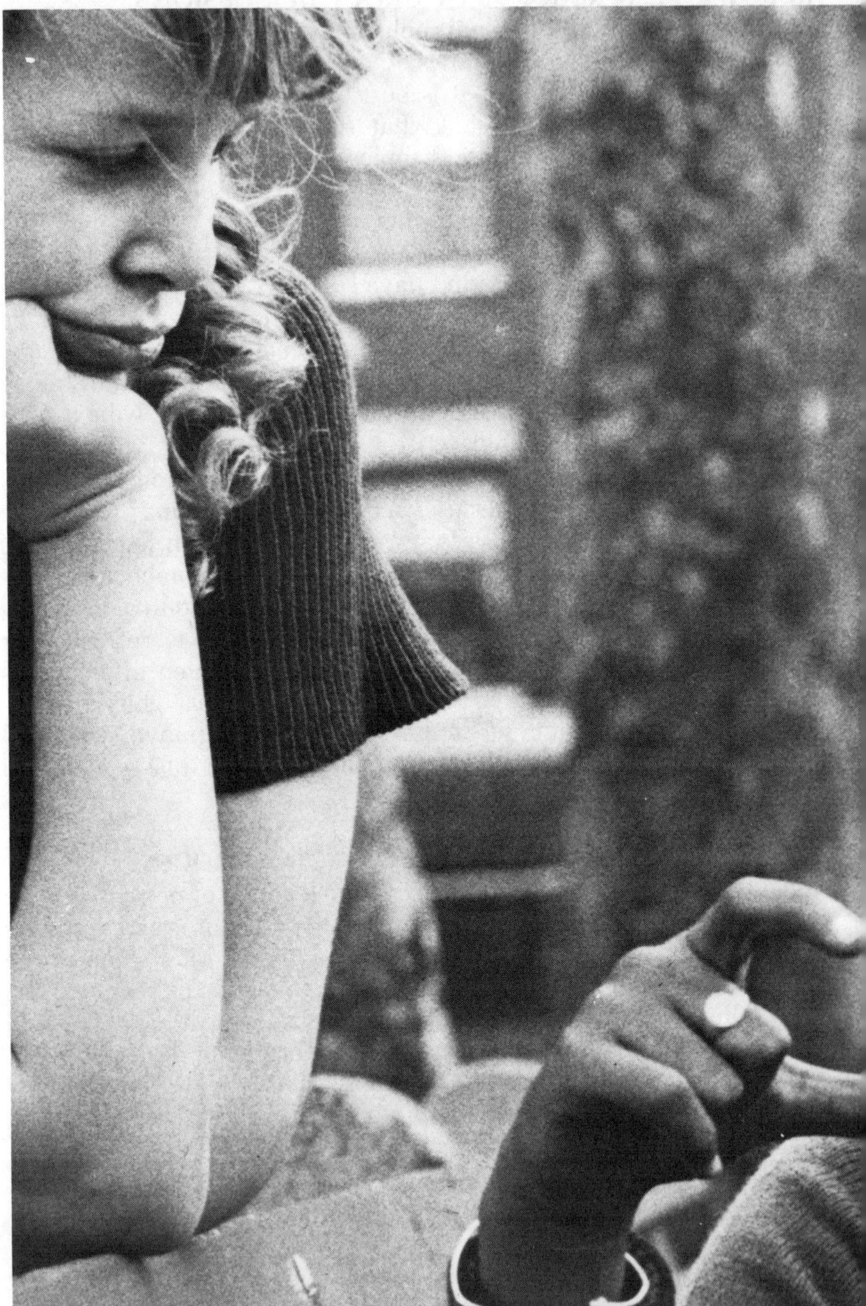

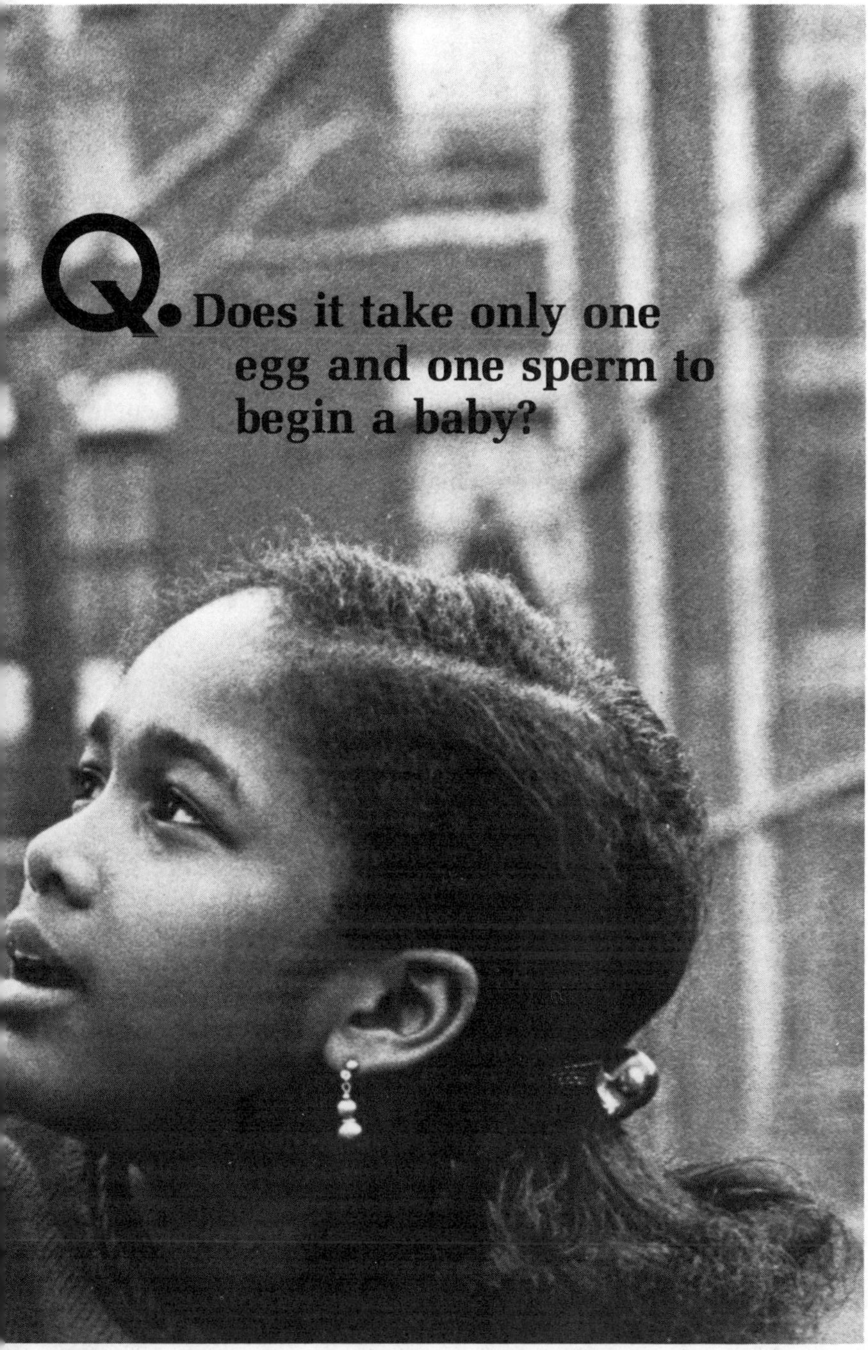
Q. Does it take only one egg and one sperm to begin a baby?

CHAPTER 4

GETTING STARTED

WELL, here you are! You're sitting in a circle with nine, wide-eyed, fidgety children. You've read everything in the field of sex education you could lay your hands on, you've practiced your new vocabulary, you're ready to embark on your career as a sex educator — and you have the strong impression that this may be the longest half hour of your life! Cheer up! We think you've passed the first test for successful discussion leaders: You're feeling what the children are feeling — you're involved!

But that's not much consolation, is it? Feeling involved may be well and good but what do you actually do now? First, relax, take a deep breath and smile. Then, look the group over. Are the children sitting in a circle? Are there some unoccupied chairs interspersed with those being used? Are one or two of the youngsters sitting slightly apart from the others, or is there one almost in your lap? If there are extra chairs, ask the children to remove them and close the circle; if some children are outside the circle, ask them to move in. These simple procedures have a twofold purpose — they immediately unite the group physically, and they further a continuous flow of conversation.

Where the children are sitting in relation to one another within the circle is not too important during this first session. But as time goes on and you continue to permit the kids to sit wherever they wish, be aware of each child's choice. The least liked child will probably sit apart from the others, not by his design, but by theirs. Good friends will not want to be separated. There most likely will be those who decide they want to sit together so they can deliberately bait one another. The shy one will be alone, even in the group, chair pushed slightly back. The one who craves affection will sit next to you. After a while, a pattern will take shape; most children will take the same seats week after week without being assigned to them. Being a careful observer of the physical relationship within the circle will assist you later in establishing group rules, while permitting the children the ultimate in verbal freedom. For instance, there will be times, when you know the group well, when it will be wise for you to seat yourself after the children have taken their places. If you have previously noted that two children sitting together are an unfortunate combination and have been a disrupting influence, you can quietly sit between them without making an issue of it. If you see that a child is continuously overactive and has trouble sitting still, you can seat yourself next to him or her — often, just a gentle hand on the child's shoulder is all that is necessary to restore calm.

When the circle is closed, we suggest that you go through a settling down procedure, before you actually start any discussion. We feel that it is always a good idea to allow a few seconds at the beginning of each session to gain the attention of the group. You can usually achieve this by simply waiting until the chatter has ceased and all eyes are on you, not saying a word, a pleasant, expectant expression of your face. This silent pause has a calming effect and relaxes everyone.

EXPLAIN THE NATURE OF THE MEETING

The kids are quiet; at last it's time to begin the heart of the program. Tell the children that they are going to meet with you for half an hour each week and that they are going to be a discussion group. Let them explain what they think a discussion is. "It's talking" or "It's saying something" are some of the responses you can expect to hear. "Fine," you say, "but what do you think we are going to talk about?" You will probably get a flood of answers ranging from "pets" and "families" to "electricity" and "science." "We'll probably talk about those things," you can assure them, "because in this group you can talk about

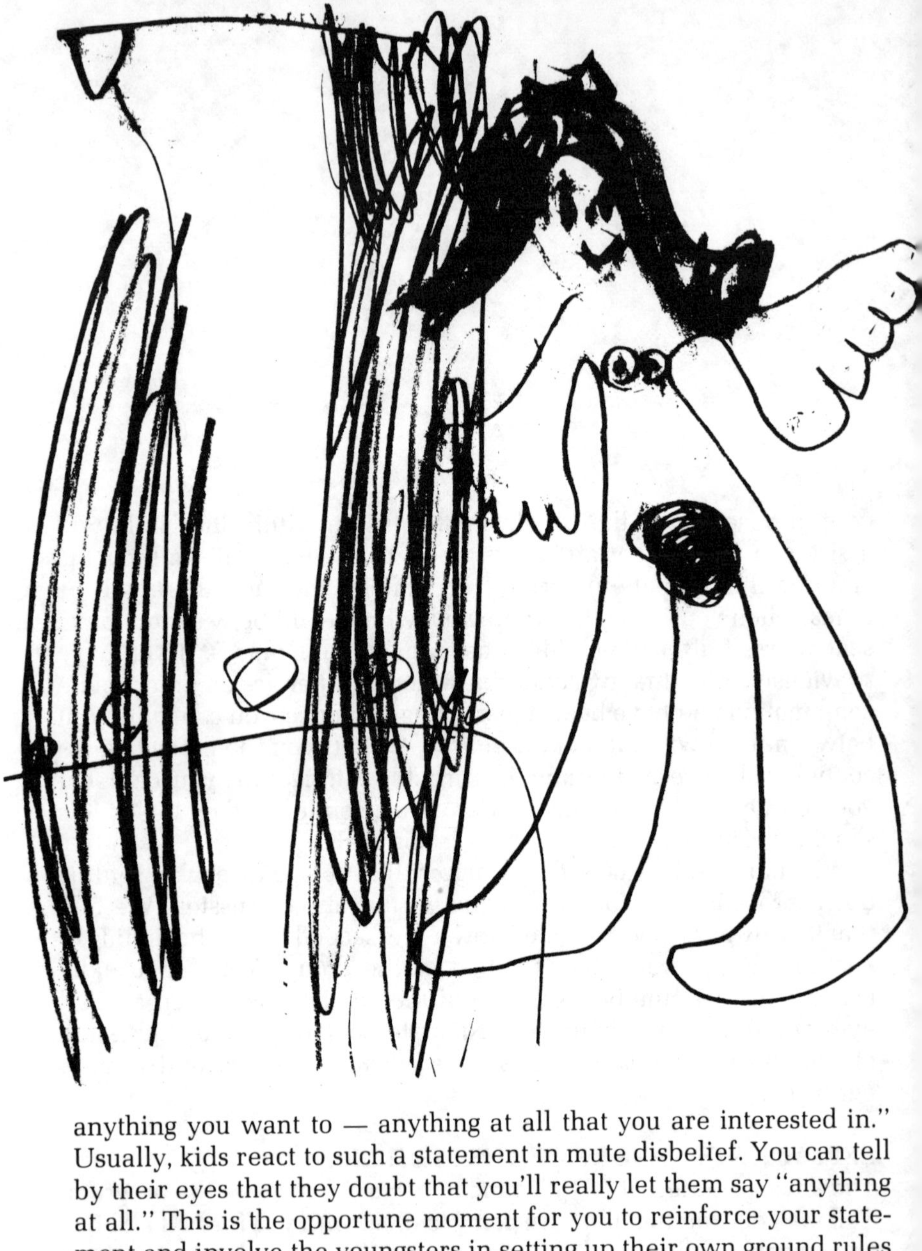

anything you want to — anything at all that you are interested in." Usually, kids react to such a statement in mute disbelief. You can tell by their eyes that they doubt that you'll really let them say "anything at all." This is the opportune moment for you to reinforce your statement and involve the youngsters in setting up their own ground rules for meetings.

You can expect to hear a barrage of suggestions, some verging on the ridiculous: "We shouldn't spit"; "We shouldn't kick or bite each other"; "We shouldn't push anyone off a chair." But you will also hear the rules that are going to make your groups successful: "We shouldn't talk when someone else is talking"; "We should take turns";

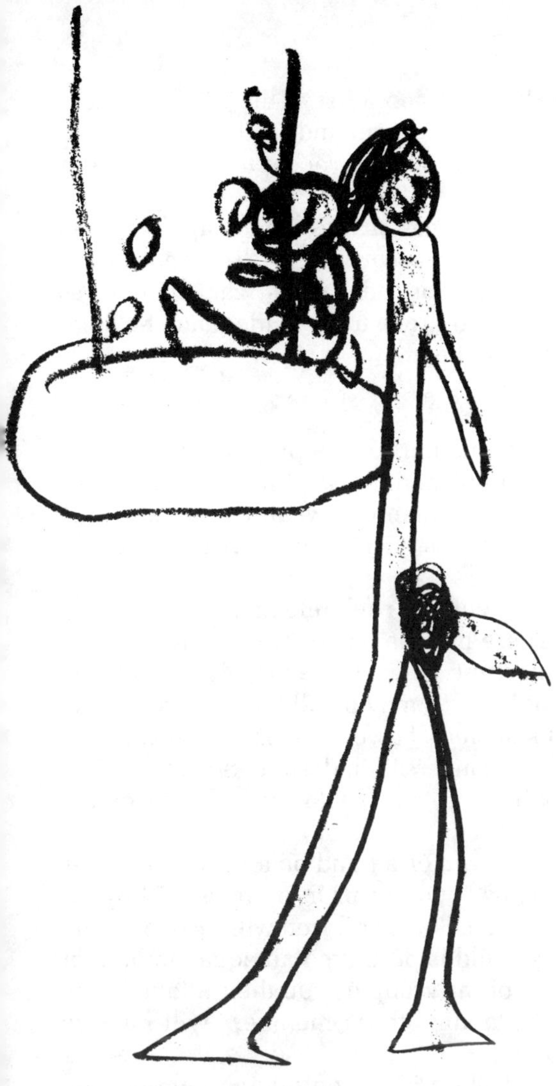

"We should listen when someone else is talking and not interrupt"; "Only one person talks at a time." Quite simply, the children will set up the basic rules for their meetings.

As the need for additional rules arises, as it most likely will, again ask the cooperation of the group in working out a fair method of controlling itself. Also ask the group to decide on consequences for people who break the rules. (In other words, have the children make a contract with you.) You will, no doubt, have to assist the group in choosing *reasonable* consequences; otherwise, you may end up with suggestions for eight or nine children to be strung up by their toenails, or to write "I will not interrupt when someone else is talking" twenty thousand times on the blackboard. Keep a list of the rules and consequences the children have decided upon, and, at the beginning of the first few meetings, ask the youngsters to repeat them to you as a means of reminding themselves.

No one set of rules and consequences always will be applicable to every group; each group will vary according to the needs of its members. Let the children decide for themselves what their rules should be, and if those rules should prove to be inadequate, be flexible and help the group to change them.

DISCIPLINE

Discipline, too, should be a flexible part of the program. With some groups you will never have to think about discipline — the children will be too interested in one another and in whatever is being discussed to misbehave. In those groups, you'll feel more like a group member than a leader.

However, all groups probably will not run quite that smoothly — at least, not in the beginning. There may be one or two youngsters in a group who continuously interrupt when someone else is talking. Group censorship of those individuals may be all that is necessary to get them in line. If that isn't sufficient, however — if a child still persists in trying to monopolize the conversation despite the obvious displeasure of his peers—it will be up to you to take charge of the situation.

Sometimes, just a glance from you or a hand on a child's shoulder will remind him that he is talking out of turn. Or, perhaps, calling out his name may be all that is needed. Some children will respond quite well if you mention that each child is permitted an equal amount of time to talk; if some members of the group use up their allotted time interrupting while others are talking, those members will have to forego their turns.

If, despite these measures, a child keeps on talking, remind him that everyone wants to have an opportunity to talk and that everyone wants to be listened to — if he can't be more considerate of other people's feelings, he will have to sit *outside* the circle. Make it clear to him that he cannot participate in the discussion while sitting outside the circle, but make it equally clear that he can re-enter the circle any time he feels ready to abide by the rule, "Only one person talks at a time."

While a child is sitting outside the circle, his space within should be left open. Tell the group that you feel that each child has something of value to contribute — you hope the child who is momentarily on the outside will soon be able to exert sufficient self-control and come back and close the circle. Leaving the space open, to be filled at the child's option, is a face-saving device for him. Because most children will not want to give up their opportunity to talk, their stay outside the circle will usually be a limited one.

If even this measure does not accomplish the desired result (as it won't in some cases), you may have to tell the child that if his disturbing behavior continues, he will not be permitted to attend the next meeting. More often than not, just telling a child that he will have to miss a meeting will cause him to settle down, because most children really look forward to every meeting. However, if he continues to test you, follow through and don't allow him to meet with his group the following week.

Occasionally, you will find yourself confronted with an entire group (or a sizable portion of a group) who just can't seem to sit still or keep from talking among themselves long enough to get a discussion going. Obviously, you cannot remove the whole group from the circle, and although you may decide to disband the meeting, this certainly isn't something that you would want to do on a regular basis. How, then, do you deal with this group? We offer several suggestions which have worked for us:

1. Every so often, during the course of a meeting, ask a question, such as, "Who remembers what Jimmy told us a few minutes ago?" or "What was Karen talking about a little while ago?" This serves a twofold purpose: it gives Jimmy and Karen a feeling of importance; it also provides all the children with increased motivation to listen when others are talking, so that they will be able to answer your question the next time.

2. Start a session by asking who can remember some of the things that were discussed the previous week, or end a session by asking about the subjects that were discussed that day. This technique also gets children into the habit of really listening, and it will give you a good indication of the topics that were of particular interest to each child.

3. Make it a point to give positive reinforcement to those children who have been especially alert listeners each week. Praise them for their ability to recall details. Hopefully, the others will also seek positive feedback from you by following the examples set by the more attentive members of the group. This approach generally accomplishes much more than that of continuously singling out or finding fault with those who misbehave.

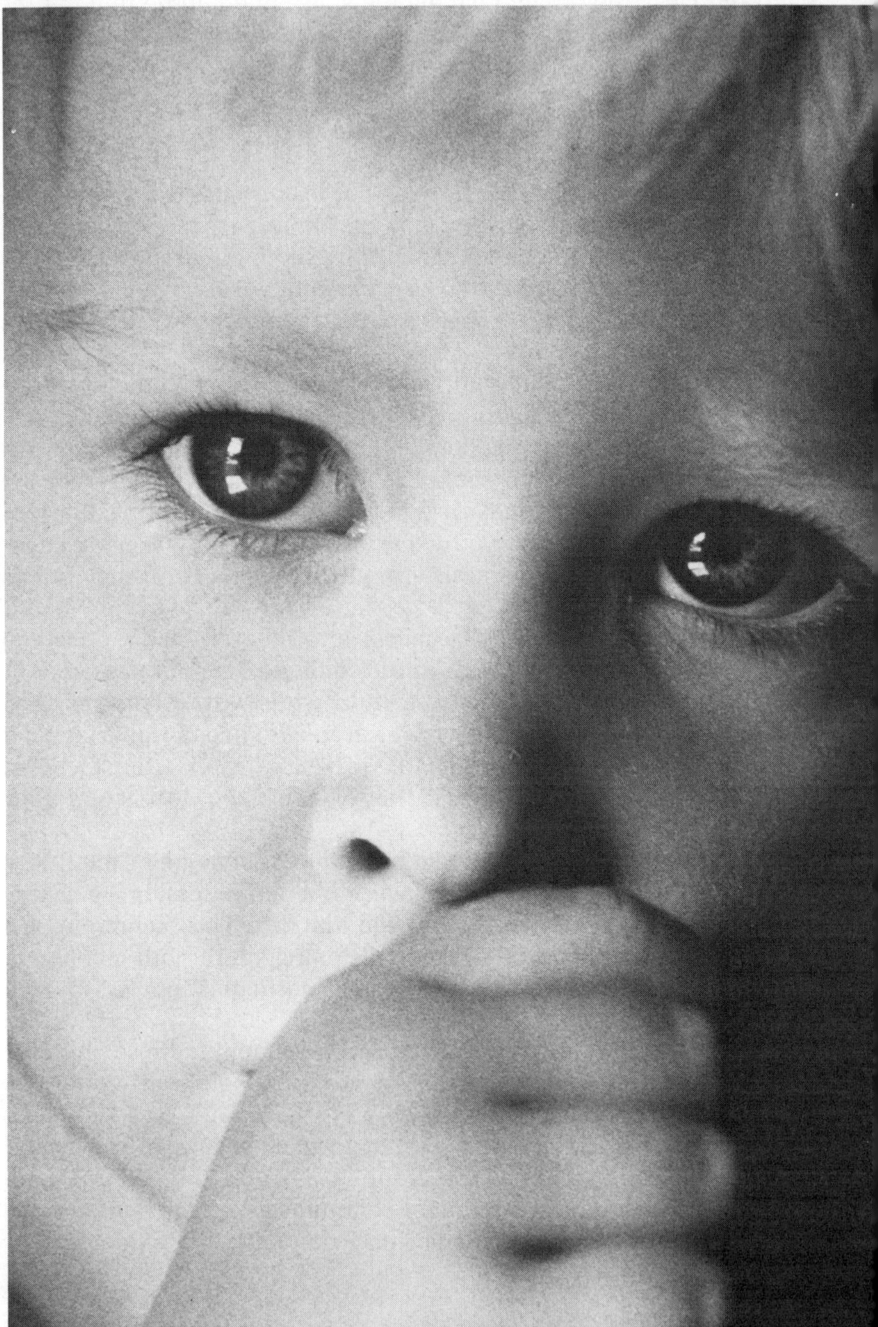

Q. Why does a mommy have to go to the hospital to have her baby?

CHAPTER 5

HOLDING DISCUSSIONS

WHEN WE first began teaching sex education, we thought that the children in our groups would be able to speak out whenever they felt like it, just as adults do when they are engaged in a discussion. The result was chaos! In a relatively short time, we knew that the idea was not going to work. The children also made it clear that they preferred to raise their hands and let the discussion leader select the speaker; this system allowed everyone to have an equal number of turns to talk, if they wished.

In order to make certain that every child does have an equal chance to talk, tell the group that everyone will be offered turns during each session, but that no one is under any obligation to speak unless he or she wants to. No child should have a second turn until all members of the group have been offered a first turn. Be sure to point out that if someone does not choose to speak when given the opportunity, you will call on that person before you call on anyone else, should he have something he wants to say later on.

The shy child, in particular, benefits from this technique. He may not have the courage to raise his hand or to speak when you call on him the first time, but he may choose to do so later. If he cannot bring himself to enter the conversation week after week, and the others mention that he never talks, be sure to reassure him that he is a good listener and that he need not speak if he doesn't feel in the mood; point out to the group as a whole that good listeners are as important to a discussion group as good talkers.

Eventually, you will probably find that even the very quiet child who never, or almost never, participates in classroom discussions, will begin to talk within the small group setting; the feeling of intimacy that exists, accompanied by a lack of demands or pressures, tends to have a comforting, confidence-building effect.

CHILDREN'S DISCUSSIONS

The first discussions of young children who are permitted to select their own subject matter are apt to be totally unlike the adult concept of a discussion. Usually, when we think of a discussion, we think of a group of individuals speaking about one topic, each contributing their ideas about that topic and finally coming to a definite conclusion.

Your students' initial discussions, however, will be somewhat different, particularly because your primary goal is to create something rather intangible: a relaxed atmosphere in which a feeling of trust and rapport develops between you and the children and among the children themselves. As the children introduce topics, try to guide them into areas that will hold the interest of the whole group, stimulating a flow of viewpoints and ideas and encouraging the children to think for themselves. In order to insure that they can talk about anything that they want to, however, you will have to go along with the group; if the children flit from topic to topic, you will have to curb your desire to continue along one vein of thought or to make a point.

Curbing your natural tendencies may be frustrating in the beginning; you will probably be tempted to encourage the children to finish what they started, and to bring the conversation to a logical conclusion. You will probably feel the need to "achieve," and to observe concrete results. Bear in mind, however, that you are working in an area in which you are not required to give tests or grades — you will not be under any pressure to cover a certain amount of material in a certain amount of time, so RELAX!

THE GENERAL DISCUSSIONS

When you're ready to begin a discussion, try a leading question as an icebreaker; direct it to the child who was most vocal when you were establishing your guidelines. "Did you have a good summer?" "Do you have any brothers or sisters?" "Do you have any pets at home?" "How do you like first grade (second grade, etc.)?" Usually, after the first child answers, hands begin to go up and the others volunteer information about the subject. However, in the event that your initial questions don't evoke much of a response, begin talking about yourself. You may not be able to finish more than one or two sentences, because once you start speaking about yourself, the children will almost certainly want to talk about themselves.

In subsequent meetings, you probably will find that you need say no more than an interested, "What's new?" or "How's everything?" The hands will shoot up in the air and your only concern will be to decide who should talk first. Vary your method of doing this. If only one hand is up, you have no problem. But if most of the children want to talk, try alternative ways of selection. Move clockwise or counterclockwise around the circle. Go back and forth across the circle, starting with the child on your left and then cross to your right. You can choose the child sitting opposite you and go clockwise, counterclockwise or back and forth across the circle starting with that child. You can make a game of the process; write down a number between one and fifteen and let the child who comes closest to that number go first. Or you can ask a boy to choose a girl and she in turn can choose a boy, or let them call on whomever they want. We do not use these last two methods very often, because the same children tend to be left out each time. However, if you do have the children call on one another occasionally, pay particular attention to their selections — they'll give you considerable insight into each member's social status within the group.

GUIDING THE DISCUSSIONS

Your first five or six meetings will probably deal with general topics, such as pets, movies, television programs, birthday parties, vacations, etc. These initial discussions are very important, since they set the tone and lay the foundation for your future relationship with the children. One way that you can make the first meetings more interesting, meaningful and involving is by listening carefully for key words and phrases which can serve as focal points for discussions. Here are some of the topics children often introduce during this "testing" or warm-up period, and some sample questions you can ask that will start discussions.

Birthdays: What is a birthday?

Why do we have birthdays?

How do you feel about growing up?

Would you rather be a child or an adult?

What is your favorite way to celebrate your birthday?

What was the nicest thing anyone ever did for your birthday?

What was the nicest thing you ever did for someone else's birthday?

When was the happiest birthday you remember?

When was the unhappiest birthday you remember?

Families: What is a family?

What is a grandfather, grandmother, brother, sister, aunt, uncle, cousin?

What do mothers do?

What do fathers do?

Does every family have the same number of people?

Do you have chores to do at home? What are they?

Do you get paid for doing chores? If you didn't get paid, would you still do them?

How does your family manage when your mother or father is sick or when one of them is away from home for a long period of time?

What is your position in the family (first, second, third child, etc., or only child)?

How do you feel about your position in the family? Would you rather be the oldest, the youngest? Why?

Would you prefer to be a member of a big family or a small family? Why?

What kinds of things does your family do together?

Why do most children in the same family fight so much, and what suggestions do you have for settling arguments?

What things do you have to share at home and what things are yours alone?

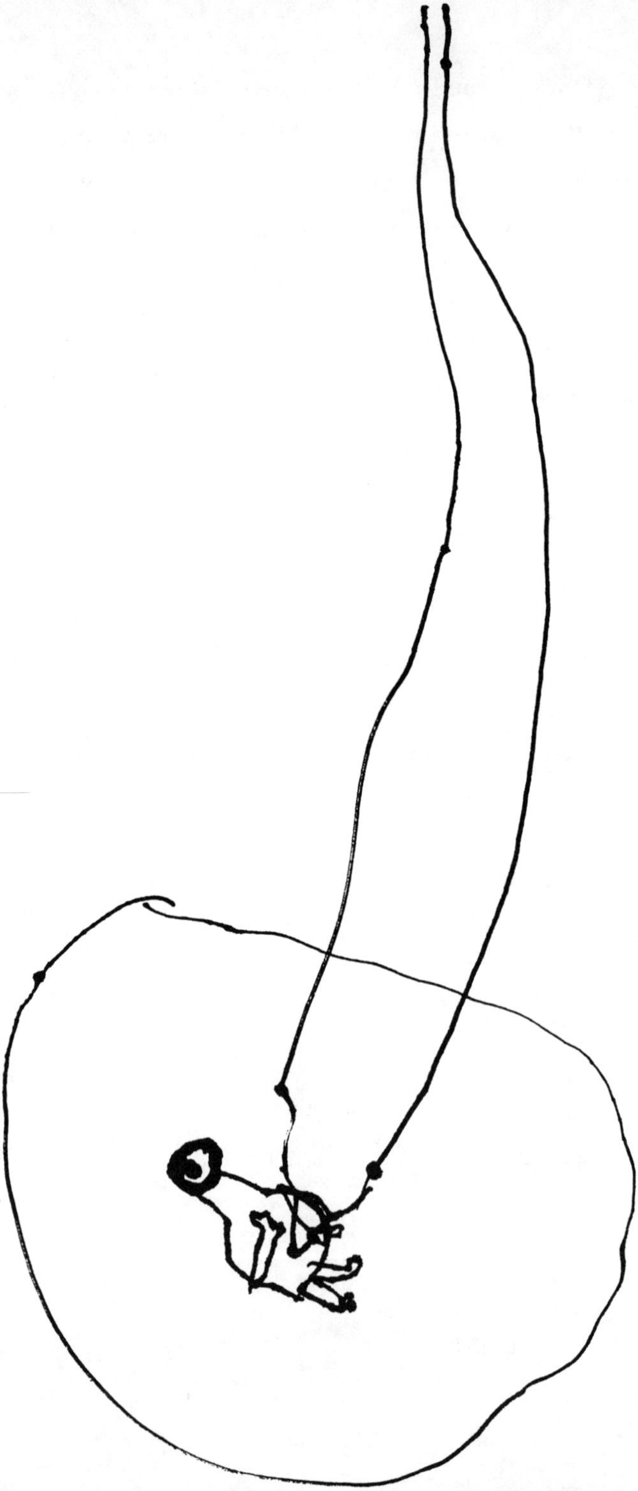

Do both your parents work and how do you feel about that?

What is a wedding?

Why do people get married?

Do you think you will want to get married when you grow up?

Pets: Do you have any pets at home? If so, how do you take care of them?

Have you ever had to give up a pet? Why? How did you feel about giving it up?

Have you ever had a pet that died?

How can you tell when an animal or a person is dead?

What is a funeral? Have you ever been to a funeral?

How do you feel when something or someone you love dies?

What would the world be like if no one ever died?

Vacations: What was your favorite vacation?

If you could do anything you wanted to during a vacation, what would that be?

If you stay home during a vacation, how do you keep busy?

School: What do you like best about school?

What don't you like about school?

If you could make new rules for your school, what would they be?

Has anything happened in school lately that made you feel very happy? Has anything happened that made you feel unhappy?

Friends: What kind of people do you like to have as your friends?

What do you like most about your best friend?

What does it mean to be a friend?

How can you make new friends?

Television: What are your favorite television programs?

Are you allowed to watch as much television as you want, or are you only permitted to watch certain programs, or watch at certain times?

What happens if several members of your family want to watch different programs at the same time?

These are some of the first topics that children usually discuss during the getting acquainted period. After a few weeks, however, you will probably notice a subtle change in their choice of topics. They will begin to talk about subjects that have to do with feelings and are of a slightly more personal nature. This is a sign that they are beginning to trust you. They will mention fears and fantasies, problems and concerns, death, injuries, accidents, illnesses, operations, deformities, divorces, etc. You may not be aware of it at the time, but by giving them the freedom to discuss subjects dealing with all of their interests, questions and concerns about the world around them, you are paving the way for the introduction of sex.

WHEN SHOULD THE TOPIC OF SEX BE INTRODUCED?

The humanistic approach to sex education is based upon the belief that sex education should be a gradual, spontaneous and continuous process which should be introduced *when the children indicate that they are ready,* not when a teacher or a curriculum guide indicates that they should be ready. Your groups will let you know that they are ready to discuss sexual topics in the same manner that they start all of their discussions — by bringing up the topics themselves. For example, in the middle of a conversation about food, a child may suddenly mention that his mother "is getting very fat 'cause she's going to have a baby." If others in the group are interested, they will turn to the child (or to you) and ask a question, such as, "Where's the baby now?" or "How come a lady gets so fat when she's going to have a baby?" or "How does a mommy get her baby out?" If the children are not ready, they will quickly change the subject.

HELPING SEX EDUCATION TO HAPPEN

If there is no response from a group when a sexual topic is brought up, or if you have a group that takes much longer than others to get started, there are ways you can *help* sex education to happen. One way is to listen again for key phrases, just as you always should do. When the child mentions the exciting news about his expectant mother (or aunt or older sister), you may want to ask a leading question, such as, "Where is the baby now?" or "How big do you suppose the baby is now?"

The group's reaction to your question will indicate whether or not you should pursue the subject further. If the children immediately try to answer the question or if they urge you to supply the answer, you should feel free to continue in that vein. If they are not interested, they will either remain silent or they will tune you out by shifting to another topic. Some may even go so far as to say, "Do we have to talk about this?" or "Can I talk about something else? This is boring." Their unwillingness to pursue sexual topics at this particular time is no reflection on your ability to teach sex education. It usually only means that the group needs more time. (Sometimes, however, the group, or some children in it, feel threatened by rather than disinterested in sexual topics, so it's a good idea to find out the reason for the silence or change of subject.) Keep in mind that in a few weeks or months, the same group may be much more receptive to the same kind of question.

HOW MUCH AND HOW OFTEN?

In a sex education program in which discussions are based upon a child's need for answers when the child expresses that need, each group will vary in the amount of information it wants. Some groups will spend week after week engaged in conversations of a sexual nature, until all of their questions have been answered — it may take forever (or so it will seem to you) for others to hold even the most basic discussions. You will eventually discover that the frequency with which children pursue sexual topics will often reflect the maturity of the group; the less mature children will take longer to reach the sex discussion stage; and the more mature will come to this point sooner, asking more sophisticated questions. Always be sensitive to the fact that when children have had enough information or feel uncomfortable with what you are discussing, they will change the subject — follow their lead, regardless of what your feelings may be at the time.

WHAT TO EXPECT FROM THE CHILDREN

When children finally bring up the subject of sex, you may be surprised by the behavior of the group. Some youngsters won't blink an eye and will react as though nothing more significant or more unusual than the daily milk count is taking place. They can be involved in a very technical discussion about how the male and female sex cells unite and divide, and, a few minutes later, they can become equally involved in a conversation about yesterday's ball game.

Other groups of children will giggle, blush and almost fall off their chairs when the word "sex" is mentioned. Older children who have never before talked about sex within a school setting will be even more nervous and embarrassed than younger children. This is certainly natural and understandable — these children have had more years to acquire the inhibitions that promote this kind of reaction.

Don't allow nervous or unexpected reactions to discourage you. Let the children know, as often as necessary, that you understand how they feel; let them know, too, that sex is a respectable topic of conversation, because it is a respectable (and acceptable) part of life. By calmly helping them through the first embarrassing moments, the tenseness should gradually fade away and the kids will be able to deal with the subject in a more mature, relaxed manner.

WHAT STIMULATES SEXUAL DISCUSSIONS?

A child's trip to the zoo or a visit to a farm where he happened to see animals mating or giving birth, can lead to discussions on sex. The sound of a cat howling or the observation of a dog in heat can do the same. A Sunday drive in the country and the sight of animals mating in the fields can rouse a child's curiosity and he may bring his questions to school the following day.

Any experiences children may have had with household pets that gave birth may prompt them to ask questions about sex. Most children are very much interested in learning about and comparing how different animals reproduce. When a child mentions that his dog or cat had babies, ask if others in the group have seen animals being born. If they have, they may want to share their experiences with the group and an interesting and informative lesson on reproduction will take place.

A child may tell about an excursion to a county fair and his delight at the sight of a sow and her piglets. A discussion on breast-feeding is a natural extension of this story.

When a child announces that he has received a new puppy, ask him if it is male or female. Young children, especially those who come from a household where all of the youngsters are of one sex, often do not know the differences between males and females.

Raising animals in your classroom — gerbils, mice, guinea pigs, rabbits, guppies — and permitting the children to care for them, is a fine way for you to introduce your students to the reproduction process. An incubator with fertilized eggs will also provide the kids with an invaluable learning experience. Such projects will make it easier and natural to discuss reproduction in a later group meeting.

THE MASS MEDIA ALSO STIMULATES DISCUSSIONS ABOUT SEX

Television programs will be responsible for many discussions about sex. A child may tell the group that he saw a play on TV about an unmarried woman who had a baby. Another child may mention having watched a medical program dealing with venereal disease or a documentary about homosexuality. Several children in a group even may have witnessed the birth of a baby on an educational TV show.

Some children may ask about abortions because they followed the story line of a soap opera during a vacation or while they were sick in bed. Prostitution, rape and even indecent exposure are now fairly commonplace themes for prime time television plays and movies. Commercials advertising bras, sanitary napkins and remedies for irregularity can raise questions in the minds of young children.

Even though many such programs and commercials are shown during early evening hours, when children are still awake, the subject matter and the way it is presented are usually too difficult for most children to comprehend. Since they may not feel comfortable about discussing with their parents what they have seen, they may very well bring their questions and concerns to you and the discussion group.

Even newspaper and magazine articles are responsible for many discussions on sex, particularly among older children who read about sexual assault, rape and sexual deviation, as well as about birth control, the Pill and abortion. For younger children, a magazine photograph of a mother dog and her pups, posted in the classroom, can lead to a discussion about like producing like. A newspaper clipping which talks about quintuplets or Siamese twins can lead easily into conversations about multiple births or birth defects. A magazine picture showing a newborn or a mother holding her baby can also prompt the children to start talking about sex.

Children have questions and concerns about what they read, see and hear all around them — they have a need to talk about these questions and concerns, and they will talk about them if given the opportunity. Once they realize that their questions about sex will not meet with anger, raised eyebrows or ridicule, they will feel no hesitancy about bringing them to you and the discussion group to be answered.

Q. Why does the doctor slap the baby on the rear end after it's born?

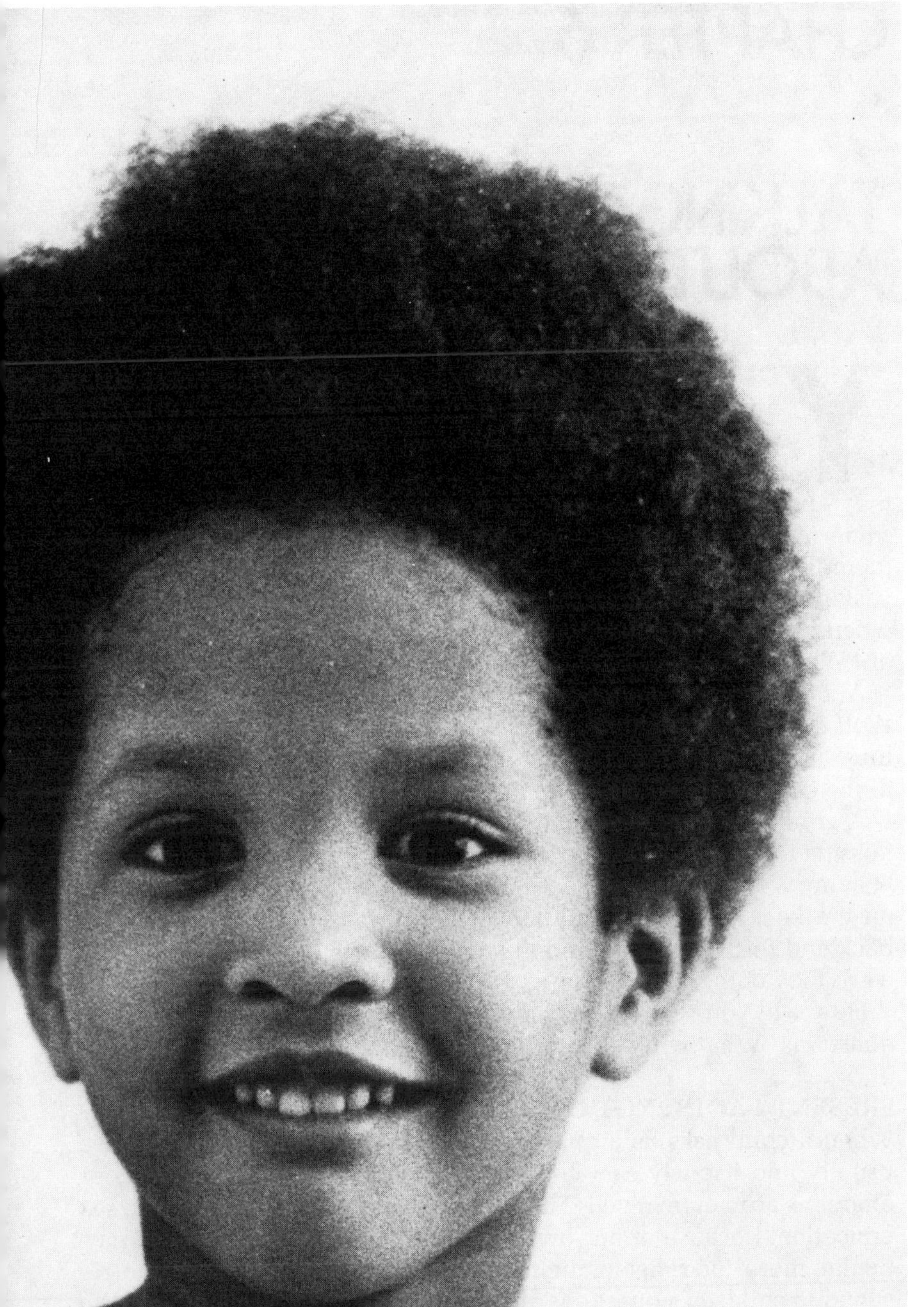

CHAPTER 6

TALKING TO CHILDREN ABOUT SEX

YOUR SMALL GROUP meetings will provide children with an opportunity to acquire correct factual information, not only about reproduction and childbirth, but about the changes that will be taking place within their own bodies as they approach puberty. The kids will want to ask questions — and some of their questions will come at times when you least expect them. For example, a group may be involved in a discussion about yesterday's softball game between the fourth and the fifth graders, when a child will suddenly ask, "What does the word 'rape' mean?" or "Why do some women want to have abortions?"

Another group may be arguing about whether *Dracula and the Wolf Man* or *Frankenstein's Revenge* was the most frightening movie they ever saw, when someone will say, "I read in the paper that a nine-year-old girl had a baby. That isn't possible, is it?"

A group of first graders may be engrossed in a conversation about missing teeth and the "tooth fairy" and all of a sudden you may hear, "On my way home from school yesterday, I saw a big black dog climb on the back of a small gray and white dog, and they were moving back and forth real fast. I didn't know what they were doing — what *were* they doing?"

How will you react when suddenly confronted with these kinds of questions? What will you do? What will you say?

PRESENT FACTS, NOT OPINIONS

When a child asks us a question about mathematics or science, we usually find it fairly easy to give an objective answer, because our emotions are not involved. This, however, isn't always the case in sex education. Because of our own upbringing, because of our own particular moral or religious beliefs, we may be sorely tempted to respond to children's questions about sex with more than just facts. We may attempt in subtle — and sometimes not so subtle — ways to influence children's attitudes and feelings about sex, so that they correspond with our own way of thinking.

Let's say, for example, that a child asks, "Can a woman have a baby if she isn't married?" — a question, by the way, that is frequently asked by second, third and even fourth graders. Obviously, there is only one correct answer — a simple "Yes." But, depending upon our own backgrounds and philosophies, we may feel that we have to embellish that simple answer. Those of us who were taught that sexual relations between unmarried people are wrong may feel compelled to answer the question something like this: "Yes, it's possible for a woman to have a baby if she isn't married, but she *shouldn't*" or "It isn't a very good idea" or "It's very difficult for a woman to raise a child without a husband."

Those of us, on the other hand, who have a more open attitude toward sex may be inclined to answer the question this way: "Yes, a woman certainly *can* have a baby if she isn't married and there's nothing wrong with it" or "In today's society, a woman can raise a child by herself with little difficulty" or "If a woman really wants to have a baby, she should have one, regardless of whether or not she is married."

Because of our personal views, some of us may find it difficult to stick to the facts when children ask us questions about such issues as abortion or birth control. Instead of just explaining what the terms mean, we may feel it necessary to let the children know our beliefs — but it is neither the role nor the right of a teacher to try to impose her value system on her students. The teacher's job is to *teach* not *preach*.

WHAT SHOULD YOU DO WHEN CHILDREN ASK FOR YOUR OPINION?

If you are meeting with older children, there will undoubtedly be times when they will ask for your opinion on a subject. A youngster may turn to you and say, "Do you think it's right for people to have sexual intercourse before they are married?" or "Don't you think it's awful for a pregnant woman to kill her baby by having an abortion?"

We suggest that when you are asked such questions, you refer the question back to the child who asked it, and then to the group for an interchange of ideas and opinions. If the child still persists in trying to pin you down, you can say, "I don't think it would be fair for me to answer that question. My answer might influence your thinking, and I would prefer that you think for yourself and draw your own conclusions." This is your privilege — the same privilege, of course, that should be granted to every child in the group.

Some teachers — especially beginning teachers — seem to feel that if they don't answer every question every child asks, they are failing the children in some way, or that they will lose respect in the eyes of the classroom. It goes without saying that if a child asks you a question requiring a factual answer and you aren't sure of your facts, you should postpone an answer until you have had a chance to look up the information. But there will also be occasions when you should not answer a question simply because you *choose* not to.

Children sometimes ask inappropriate questions about sex. After learning about sexual intercourse, for example, a child may turn to you and say, "Have *you* ever had sexual intercourse?" or "How often do you have sexual intercourse?" After a discussion on birth control has taken place, some of the children may want to know whether you use a birth control device, or, more specifically, what type of device. When questions such as these are asked, all you need say is, "That is a question we don't ask other people. It's too personal."

There may be other times when children ask questions which make you feel uncomfortable — questions about sexual deviation or perhaps about the details of a particularly bizarre sex crime. In that circumstance, you certainly have the right, just as the children do, to say, "I would rather not answer that question because talking about it makes me feel uncomfortable." Children must learn to be sensitive to a teacher's feelings, just as she must learn to be sensitive to theirs.

Occasionally, a child will ask a question that causes other children in the group to feel uncomfortable, or that deals with a matter beyond their comprehension. If you feel that the question should be answered privately, arrange to meet with the child at another time.

GIVE SHORT, SIMPLE ANSWERS

When a child asks you a question, you may be inclined to tell him more than he needs to know or even wants to know. In your eagerness to carry out your responsibilities, you may have a tendency

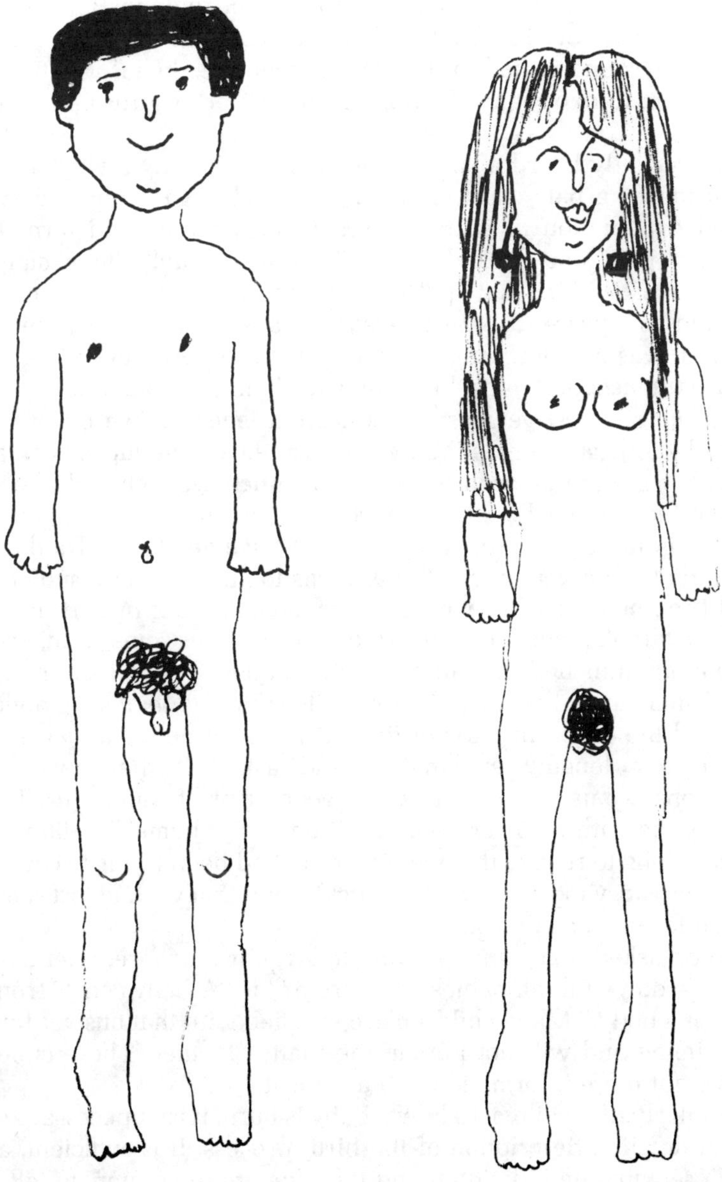

to overexplain. If your answer to a math or science question is too complicated for a child to understand, chances are that he will merely forget what you have told him until he is capable of grasping the principles involved, and no harm will have been done. But when you give a child a very involved explanation to a question about sex, one that is too sophisticated for him to comprehend, the information may cause him to experience feelings of discomfort, confusion and even fear.

We recently heard a six-year-old ask his "Family Living" teacher what makes a baby start to grow. The teacher gave him a very detailed explanation of sexual intercourse and the child turned extremely pale and looked sick. "That isn't true!" he exclaimed. "You're just making that up!" Then he ran out of the room. This child, like most six-year-olds, was not ready to absorb that kind of information; he was obviously told too much, too soon. And even though he refused to accept it, most likely he wasn't able to forget it.

During our first year as sex education teachers, we always tape recorded our group meetings. When we played the tapes back after school, we were amazed to hear how much we sounded like high school biology teachers lecturing to our students (who happened to be first graders!) before a final exam. We seemed to be afraid that if we didn't tell a youngster all there was to know about a subject the first time he asked, we would never have another opportunity.

For example, when a child asked where babies come from, we immediately launched into an explanation about sex cells in the male and female and about how the two cells unite and then keep dividing until all the different parts of the baby are formed. After we completed our lengthy explanation and asked if there were any questions, we usually heard: "Can I get a drink of water?" or "I have to go to the bathroom" or "When is it time to go home?" It didn't take us very long to realize that we obviously had been trying to cover too much territory too soon and too quickly, and that we had lost some of the children along the way.

When asked that same question today, our response, after asking, "Where do *you* think babies come from?" is "A baby comes from its mother's body." Many children are satisfied with that answer for the time being and will not pursue the matter further. Those children who want more information will ask for it.

Similarly, if a child asks how a baby is born, it isn't necessary to go into a detailed description of the birth process. It is sufficient, after again seeking the individual and then the group opinion, to tell him that a baby comes out of a special opening between the mother's legs called the vagina. If this explanation does not satisfy him, he will indicate as much by asking additional questions.

Keeping in mind that it is much easier to add information than to take it away, try to remember to answer children's questions about sex as briefly and as simply as possible. A comprehensive list of the questions you can expect to hear from children at various grade levels, along with answers you may use as guidelines, appears in Chapter 8 of this book.

TRY TO DETERMINE WHAT A CHILD IS REALLY ASKING BEFORE ANSWERING HIS QUESTION

Surely you have heard the story about the child who said to his mother, "Mommy, where did I come from?" and, after being told the "facts of life" in great detail, remarked, "I meant, did I come from California or Connecticut?" That anecdote isn't as farfetched as it may sound, because when children ask questions, adults often assume that they are asking something much more significant than is actually the case.

A first grade teacher told us about the time a little girl came up to her desk and asked, "Teacher, how do you make a baby?" Having been caught completely unaware, the teacher quickly collected her thoughts and then explained to the child how a sperm cell fertilizes an egg cell. The little girl listened patiently and then said, "I *mean*, how do you *draw* a baby?"

To further illustrate our point, when a child asks where baby kittens come from, he may be asking what part of the mother cat's body the kittens come from, or he may be asking nothing more complicated than where does a cat usually have her babies — in the basement, under the bed, in a box?

We once heard a young boy ask his mother how a puppy "gets out," and the mother, assuming that he wanted to know about the birth process, told him all about it. As it turned out, all the child was interested in finding out was how a puppy gets out of the box he is put in right after he is born; in other words, is the puppy able to climb out by himself or does the mother dog pick him up and carry him out?

In order to prevent giving a child more information than he is able to handle at the time, it is very important to try to determine exactly what he wants to know. How can you find out? Simply by saying to him, "I'm not sure I understand what you are asking" or "Please ask that question a different way so that I'm sure I know what you mean."

RESPOND TO CHILDREN'S QUESTIONS WITH THE "WHAT DO *YOU* THINK?" TECHNIQUE

Once you have determined what it is a child really wants to know, we suggest that you ask him to answer his own question. Say to him, "What do *you* think?" or "How do *you* think such and such happens?" His answer will not only give you an indication of how much he already knows, or thinks he knows about the subject, but it will also provide you with some insight into why he has asked the question.

Sometimes a child already knows the answer to a question he asks. He may ask it because he needs reassurance of his facts, or, perhaps, because something is confusing or disturbing him. He may even be asking just to see how you will respond; he wants to know if he can come to you for honest answers to his questions. You are likely to find that some children will ask you time and again how a man and woman "make a baby," even though you have answered the question any number of times. Why do they keep asking? They ask because they find the answer so difficult to accept. "Will I have to do *that* when I grow up?" they will ask. Or "Did *my* parents do that to get me?" They will be reassured if, along with the factual information, you try to convey to them the idea that to most adults, sexual intercourse represents a natural, pleasurable expression of love. The more opportunities youngsters have to discuss their thoughts and fears, the easier it will be for them to understand, and finally to accept, the whole "incredible" concept.

HELP KIDS GET THEIR THOUGHTS AND FEELINGS INTO THE OPEN

Most of the time, when a child asks a question, it is because he really wants to know the answer. Young children are genuinely interested in learning about how a baby develops inside its mother's body, and how it is born. Older children are tremendously curious about how life begins, about what makes a baby start to grow inside its mother. And most children have many misconceptions about sexual processes, some derived on their own, some learned from other children and still others learned from adults. These misconceptions should be thoroughly explored before new information is discussed.

A child might ask, for instance, "How is a baby born?" If your response is, "How do *you* think it is born?" he will probably say, "The doctor cuts the mother's stomach open, takes the baby out and sews the stomach back together." Almost every young child we have known has had this mistaken notion of how a baby is normally born; as a result, many came to our group meetings possessing very negative feelings about childbirth, envisioning it as a terribly serious, frightening and bloody operation. It is important to give children an opportunity to get such feelings out into the open, which you can do by simply asking, "How do *you* think a baby is born?"

Similarly, when a child asks how a woman becomes pregnant and you ask him how *he* thinks it happens, you can expect to hear such responses as the following:

"It happens when a man and a woman kiss."

"A lady gets pregnant from sitting on a man's lap."

"They have to touch bellybuttons."

"A woman swallows a seed and a baby starts to grow."

"The mother goes to the doctor and he gives her some medicine that makes a baby start to grow."

"Ladies have a baby machine in their bodies. They push a button and a baby pops out."

"You go to the baby section of a department store and buy a baby."

Children have a way of putting together bits and pieces of information and coming up with conclusions that often confuse, frighten or worry them. In one of our groups, there was a child who had overheard her mother telling a friend that their dog was "in heat" so now she could become pregnant. The child concluded that becoming pregnant had something to do with hot weather; she revealed during one of our meetings that she was afraid to go outdoors in the summer for fear that she would somehow become pregnant.

Still another child, who had been told by her mother that a baby grows from a seed in the mother's stomach, admitted to us that for years she had worried about the possibility of becoming pregnant from swallowing a seed — so she refused to eat anything that contained seeds. Such are the misconceptions that children must be given opportunities to talk about.

There is one more reason for responding to children's questions about sex with "What do *you* think?" This simple technique will give you a chance to collect your thoughts and to decide how you can best answer a question. Sometimes, the first answer that comes to your mind is not the most appropriate one; if you give yourself just a few moments to reflect, you will probably think of something more suitable to say. We have been answering children's questions about sex for many years, but there are still times when we are caught completely off guard — we really aren't certain we know how to answer a question or, in fact, if we should answer it at all. Referring the question back to the child will give you the extra time you may need to decide which approach to take.

ENCOURAGE CHILDREN TO ANSWER EACH OTHER'S QUESTIONS

We have found that children often learn more willingly and more enthusiastically from one another than from an adult. We therefore

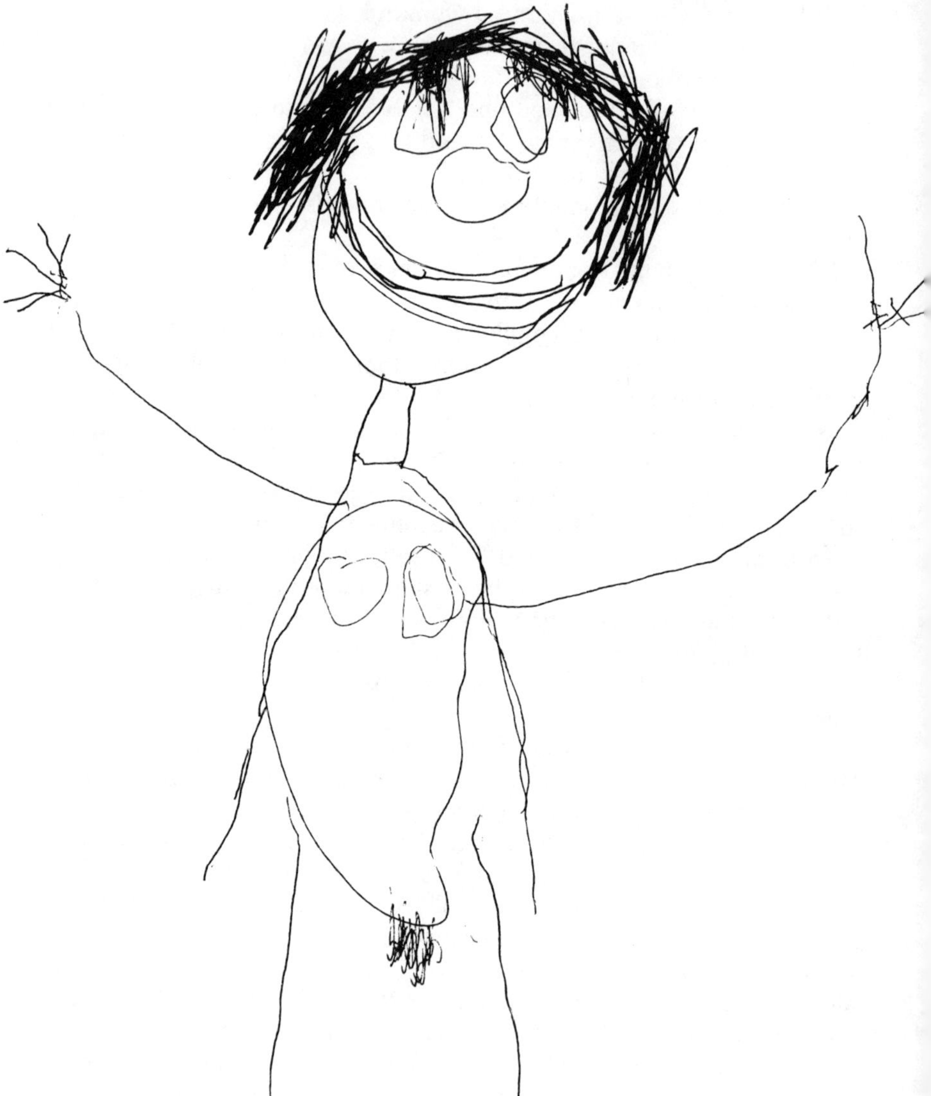

try, whenever possible, to have a child's questions about sex answered by other children in the group.

If you are fortunate, you will have in your groups at least one or two children who have already been correctly taught how a baby is conceived, develops and is born. Given the opportunity, these children usually are able to talk about what they have learned with surprising accuracy and candor; because the information is being related by another child rather than by you, an adult, the other children in the group may accept it more readily. We recall, for example, the following definitions, offered by children, which were graphic, to the point and easily understood by the other children:

"Sexual intercourse is a lot like friction. When the two parts are rubbed together, instead of a spark coming out and starting a fire, the sperms come out and start a baby."

"Afterbirth — All the insides that the baby was using come out."

"The umbilical cord is real 'womb' service."

"Intercourse is like an extension cord. The man plugs in his penis and sends the sperm cells into the uterus like a message."

Like many adults, some children are self-conscious about discussing sex-related topics — they find it difficult (and embarrassing) to use sex words and terms. Your telling children that sex can be talked about openly and without embarrassment will reassure them, but not nearly so much as hearing sex discussed by their peers. When a six-year-old hears another six-year-old use words like "uterus," "penis," "vagina" and "breasts" in the same tone of voice he would use for "finger," "toes," "ears" or "face," the child concludes that the sex-related words really are acceptable, and that he, too, can say them without feeling foolish. This will be particularly noticeable when a child who has transferred from another school joins your group during the school year. When the other children talk about sexual topics, the new child may be shocked, unaccustomed to this kind of freedom. If he laughs or makes faces or silly remarks when he hears sex terms used, the other children will quickly point out to him that he is acting "babyish" or "immature" — and this will have much more effect on the child than your telling him that his behavior is inappropriate.

A newcomer in one of our second grade groups giggled every time someone used the word "underwear." Finally, one of the boys impatiently declared, "What's the big deal about underwear? After all, we all wear it." The boy stopped laughing at that particular word, but still had a difficult time controlling himself whenever the word "penis" was said. After awhile, one of the girls gave him a very condescending look and said, "You know something — you're really weird! When you laugh at the word 'penis,' you're really just laughing at yourself. And the human body is nothing to laugh at." Such censure from the peer group finally put an end to the giggles.

WHAT IF SOME CHILDREN ARE MORE CURIOUS ABOUT SEX THAN OTHERS?

You will no doubt have groups in which some children will indicate, both by the number of questions they ask and by the nature of the questions, that they are ready to discuss sex earlier than others.

If a group has one or two children who ask questions about sex week after week while the other seven or eight children aren't the least bit interested, we suggest that you either change the two youngsters to a group that *is* interested in talking about sex or if that isn't feasible, ask them to meet with you before or after class from time to time, so that you can deal with their questions apart from the rest of the group.

If, on the other hand, you have a group of eight or nine children who frequently engage in rather mature conversations about sex, and one or two children who find it difficult to comprehend or to participate in the discussions, you really have no choice but to put the less mature children into a group in which they would feel more comfortable.

Unless you are faced with an extreme situation, however, such as the two we have just described, you needn't concern yourself too much if occasionally some of the children in a group ask more questions than others, or if some of them are interested in delving deeper than the rest of the group. We have found that more often than not, those youngsters who are not ready to absorb or are not interested in the kind of information some of the others are discussing will simply "tune out." At a later date — in a week, a month or even a year — these children probably will be ready to accept the knowledge that the others have already absorbed; then they will ask questions which other group members will be able to answer.

HOW SHOULD YOU HANDLE "SWEAR" WORDS AND "DIRTY" JOKES?

When you tell children that during the meetings they can talk about anything they want to, you can expect some of them to test you — they will try to find out if you really mean what you say. One very effective way for them to do this is by using profanity in your presence. A child may suddenly ask, "Can we use the 'f' word in here?" or he may not even ask, but simply blurt it out.

How you react at such times is of the utmost importance. If you indicate, either by word, gesture or facial expression, that you do not approve, you are telling the children that they can't really talk about *anything* they want to; you will have gone back on your word and broken a trust you worked very hard to establish.

The child who uses profanity during a group meeting generally does so for one of two reasons: (1) he wants to get a reaction from you and/or his peers; (2) he wants to find out what the word really means. In either case, we suggest that you respond in the following manner: Ask the child who used the word if he knows its meaning. If he does not, or if he pretends that he does not, ask the other group members whether they can define the word. If the answer does not come from anyone in the group, it will be up to you to supply it. Give the kids a short, simple explanation. Then help the group to think of more appropriate words which have the same meaning as the "swear" word.

If it is possible for you to do so, we also suggest that anytime a child uses a swear word, *you* repeat the word aloud. Some of the children probably will gasp, some will avert their eyes and others will giggle and squirm. After the group has had sufficient time to react, ask them how they felt when you used the word. You can expect to hear comments, such as, "Oh, you said a bad word!" or "It isn't nice to say things like that" or "If I said that, I'd get my mouth washed out with soap."

Explain that you intentionally used the word so they would understand their own feelings and the feelings of others when profanity is used. We suggest that at this point you lead the group into a discussion on why people swear — because they are angry, unhappy, surprised, etc. Certainly, we cannot expect to obliterate swear words from our children's vocabularies simply because we teach them the meanings of the words. We can hope, however, that through these discussions, children will become more sensitive to the impact swear words have on others, and that they will employ discretion in using the words.

Q. What is impotence?

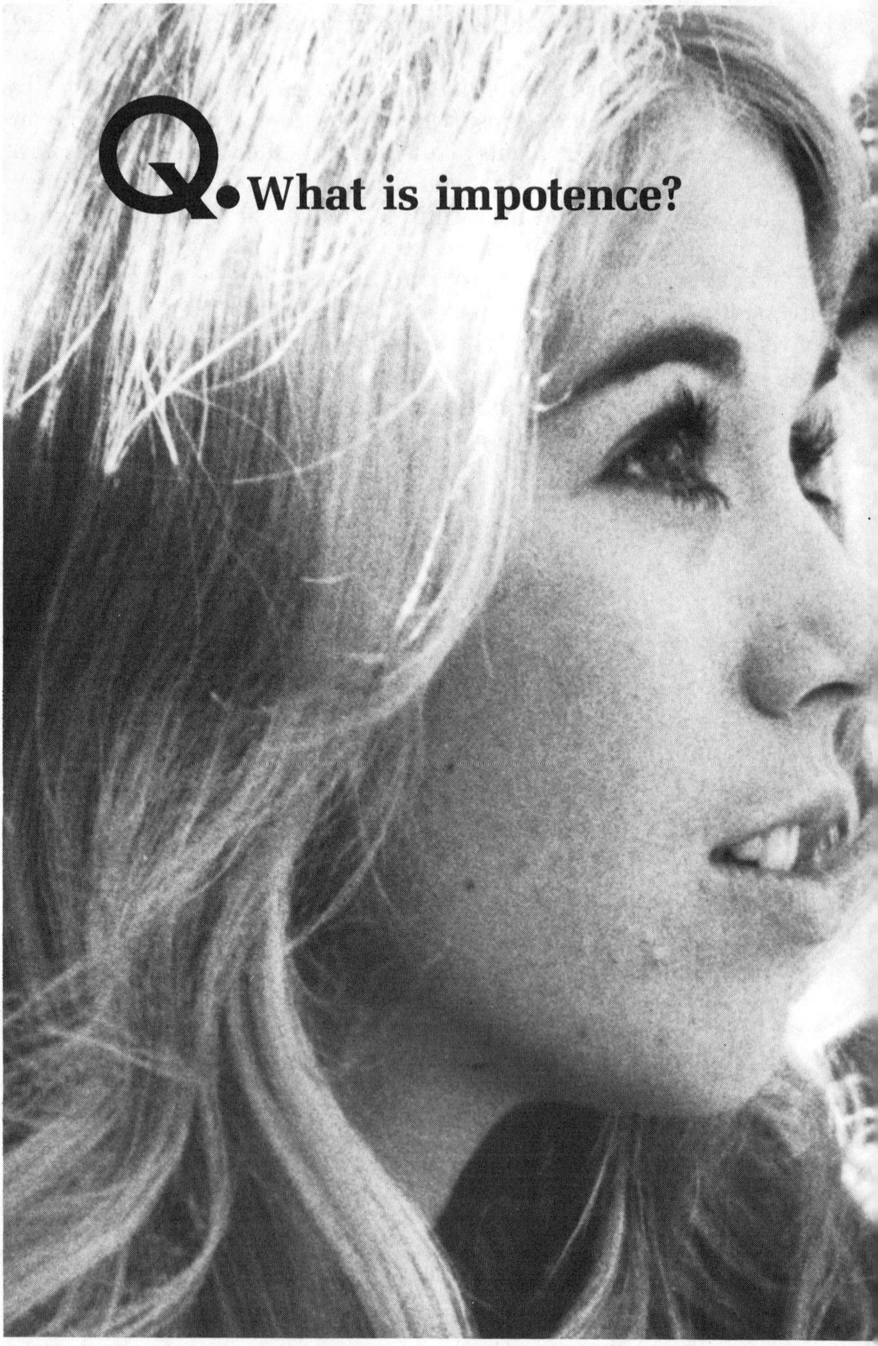

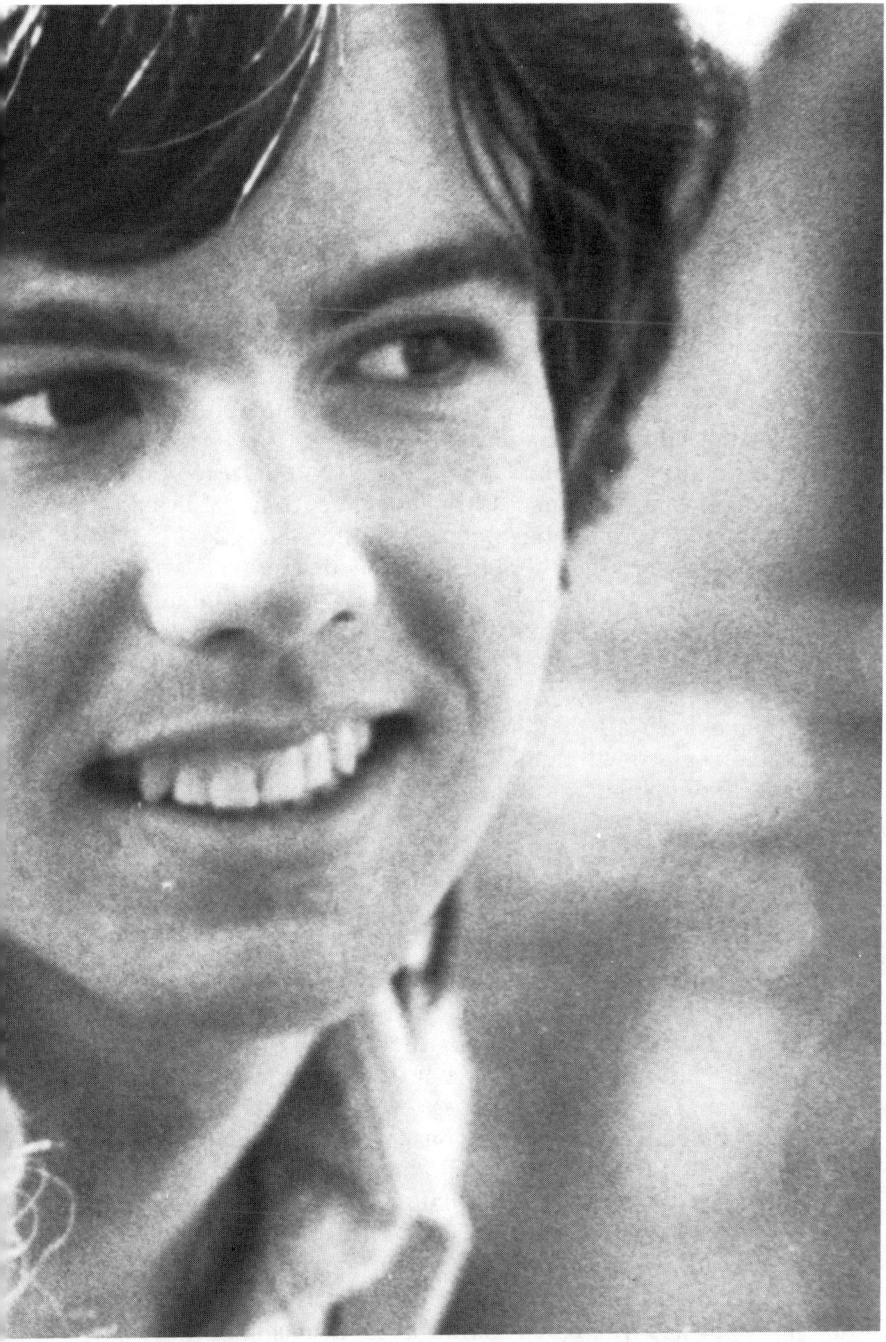

CHAPTER 7

TALKING ABOUT GROWING UP

THROUGHOUT this book, we have emphasized the point that children should receive sex education when they seem to be ready, rather than having it forced upon them according to a curriculum timetable. However, we come now to one area of sex education where it is necessary to deviate from that premise: we feel that the changes of puberty should be thoroughly covered in fifth grade (or possibly in fourth) and should be dealt with again in sixth, seventh and even eighth grade. In this way, the information will be continually reinforced. Many of your kids may have already discussed puberty by age ten, having brought it up themselves in the group meetings. If, however, they have not, it will be your responsibility to make certain that the children know about the changes that will be taking place within their bodies during the transitional period between childhood and adulthood.

THE MOST NATURAL APPROACH

There are many ways in which you can subtly initiate a discussion on puberty. Once again, listen carefully to what the children are saying; perhaps you will be able to use one of their comments as a basis for the conversation. For instance, a child might say, "I hate growing up. I wish I could be a little kid forever." You can follow up this statement by saying, "I can understand your feelings — perhaps we can all spend some time talking about what it means to grow up." Such a beginning could lead to a full discussion of growth and development.

When a child asks how old a girl has to be in order to have a baby, a discussion about menstruation and other bodily processes that begin in puberty can take place quite naturally. Even a remark about a birthday can be used to begin a discussion. "Now that you are ten (or nine or eleven) years old, have you noticed any changes in yourself or your classmates?" you might ask. Or you could say, "Now you are ten. This is the age when many children begin to change into adults."

STARTING THE DISCUSSIONS IN THE TRADITIONAL WAY

If you cannot comfortably open the discussion as the result of a child's comment, simply inform your groups that for a few weeks you will be talking about something that you feel is very important to them. It often helps to create empathy between you and the group if you tell them that even though you are now an adult, you can recall how uncertain you felt at their age. Test their readiness to become involved in a discussion of puberty by asking a few leading questions: "What do you think the word 'adolescence' or 'puberty' means?" "What changes do you think take place as children enter adolescence or puberty?" "What do we mean when we say that you have reached the age when your bodies are starting to mature?" "What are the first visible signs of physical maturity?"

HOW WILL THE CHILDREN REACT?

In some of your groups, the children will be quite open about discussing the changes of puberty. You immediately may hear, "A girl gets her period" or "A boy has wet dreams." In these instances, your job will be much easier — ask these children to explain their statements and your discussion will be under way. If there are some children who have never been told or have not absorbed facts on adolescent maturation, this will be an ideal time to ask others in the group to fill in the gaps and, with your guidance, review the information they have assimilated up to now.

Other groups will snicker, avert their eyes and be obviously embarrassed when you introduce the topic of adolescent changes. These groups will need constant reassurance that their reaction is normal, and that together you can discuss their feelings and ease the discomfort.

Regardless of how your groups respond, it is a good idea to start the discussion with simple, factual, impersonal questions; these will help to ease the way for those who find the discussion disconcerting. An example of such a question is: "Let's see if you can tell me about changes that take place when a child becomes a teenager."

Once the discussion begins, it should progress in a rather predictable way. The children probably will tell you the girls grow faster than boys during early adolescence and will be taller in eighth grade than most of the boys. However, if no one in the group mentions this, be sure to bring it up; then point out that by the time boys are in the ninth grade, most of them will begin to catch up and will continue to do so through high school. Bring out the fact that boys' voices will change and that they will develop muscles and broad shoulders. Girls' hips will broaden and breasts will develop. Both boys and girls will most likely suffer the eruptions of pimples as oil glands start to work overtime. Perspiration will begin to have an odor. Hair will appear under the arms and on boys, a few stray hairs will begin to adorn the chest, upper lip and chin. Lead your groups into discussions about normal variations in growth, physical development and personal hygiene. Many youngsters need constant reassurance that their sizes and shapes are normal — vast differences between them and their classmates often cause concern and worry. In the small group situation, kids can share their feelings of concern with their peers and find comfort in the wealth of information.

When the growth of hair is mentioned, you may notice a stir of unrest within the group. Most children at this age know about pubic hair, but are hesitant to talk about it. You may have to again assure the youngsters that discussing parts of the body that are sexual in nature is completely acceptable, and that it will help them to understand and accept the transition from child to adult.

Once the children are at ease discussing bodily changes, introduce the topics of menstruation and seminal, or nocturnal, emissions. (Seminal emissions is a subject not often touched upon in children's discussion, yet this biological change in boys can be equally as traumatic an event for them as is the onset of menstruation for girls.) We suggest that both subjects be covered during the same period because, then, neither the boys nor the girls will feel that the information being given is directed solely at them. Sharing the knowledge that members of the opposite sex are having feelings that parallel their own has a calming effect and can draw the group closer together. If, however, the youngsters are reluctant to proceed on their own, you will have to take the lead and introduce the topics.

MENSTRUATION

Keep your facts about menstruation simple and use terms that require a minimum of explanation. We explain menstruation in the following way, stating that it signifies the fact that a female is capable of having a child:

Girls are born with a uterus and two ovaries. The uterus is a pear-shaped organ or body part in the lower end of a woman's abdomen; a baby will grow here if the woman becomes pregnant. Ovaries are the two almond-shaped glands or organs on either side of the uterus. From the time a female baby is born, her ovaries contain hundreds of egg cells so small that they cannot be seen by the naked eye. Each egg cell is capable of becoming a baby if it meets with a sperm cell, which is produced by a male. The egg cells remain inactive until a girl's body changes from that of a child into that of a woman. This usually occurs some time between the ages of nine and seventeen.

When a girl reaches *the age that is right for her*, her ovaries begin to function and produce what we call "ripe," or "mature," egg cells. The first egg cell to ripen leaves one of the ovaries and starts on a journey through a narrow tube (called the Fallopian tube) which leads to the uterus. The uterus has two such tubes, one extending outward on each side, almost reaching the ovaries so they are in a convenient place to make contact with the mature egg cell. Usually, only one egg cell leaves an ovary each month and it is commonly believed that the ovaries alternate monthly, that is, one month the left ovary sends out an egg cell and the next month the right ovary does.

As the egg cell starts on the journey to the uterus, which takes between three and four days, the lining of the uterus begins to thicken and become rich with blood cells. Nature has provided this thick, soft, cushiony lining as a comfortable place in which a baby can grow if the egg cell is fertilized in the Fallopian tube. Most egg cells, however, are not fertilized, so when they reach the uterus they die, dissolve and leave the body through the vagina (another tube which leads from the uterus). The egg cell is so tiny that girls are not even aware that this is happening, because there is no pain involved.

But something else happens when an egg cell dies, of which girls *are* aware. Because the lining of the uterus will not be used to nourish and protect a baby this particular month, it disintegrates and comes loose from the wall of the uterus, leaving the body in the form of a bloody discharge (the menses). This process, called menstruation (also called a "period"), takes from three to five days and, on the average, repeats itself every 28 days. Menstruation usually continues to take place every month until a woman reaches the age of 45 to 50, at which time the ovaries cease to send out egg cells (the menopause).

During the discussions on menstruation, we recommend that you repeatedly reinforce the normalcy of individual variations — the different ages for the onset of menstruation, the different lengths and irregularity of periods, particularly when they first begin. As soon as you mention that it is possible for a nine-year-old to begin menstruating, you will probably hear, "You mean *that* could happen to *me*?" or "That means that some girls in our class already get their period." One or two of the children may even attempt to become overly personal and will start to name those who have had their first periods. This is usually done by a group member who feels threatened and seeks to draw attention away from herself. It may be necessary for you to temporarily call a halt to the conversation if this does happen, and remind the group that they can talk about the process and their own feelings, but that no one has a right to intrude on another's privacy.

Make certain that the children have sufficient time to ask questions as there will probably be many. One question in particular that probably will come up often is, "What will I do if I get my period while I'm in school?" Each school has its own method for handling this situation. Some equip their teachers with the necessary sanitary pads and belts; others have nurses or health clerks who are prepared to assist if they are needed. Whatever the procedure is in your school, make certain that you know about it and acquaint the girls with the step-by-step plan; this will keep them from panicking if the situation does occur.

SEMINAL EMISSIONS

After discussing menstruation, your groups will be familiar with the term "sperm cells," making a discussion of their production a logical next step. Remember, keep your description of the process concise, and avoid using complicated terms. Here is a simplified explanation which we have found to be effective:

Boys, too, when they reach adolescence, experience a change in their bodies which signifies that they are physically capable of fathering children. As we have said before, boys mature later than girls; they usually will show signs of puberty at about 13 or 14, although some boys may begin a year or two earlier and others a year or two later. Just as in the female, these are normal variations.

The reproductive organs in males are called the penis and the testicles, or testes. Unlike the reproductive organs of the female, they are on the outside of the body. The penis is located in the front of the body between the legs. The testicles, two tiny glands that produce sperm cells, are contained in a sac behind the penis called the scrotum. In contrast to the fact that girls are born with egg cells in their bodies, boys are not born with sperm cells in theirs. When boys reach the age of puberty, their testes start to manufacture sperm cells which are contained in a whitish, sticky fluid called semen. Usually, a boy first becomes aware of his new bodily process when he awakens one morning and discovers a small, sticky stain on his pajamas or sheets. This is nothing to become alarmed about or to feel embarrassed or ashamed about. The release of fluid is called a seminal (containing semen) or nocturnal (occurring at night) emission, or, more commonly, a "wet dream." This merely means that a boy's body is now producing sperm cells; because there was too much semen stored in his body, it overflowed and involuntarily passed out of his body through his penis.

A seminal emission takes place when a boy is asleep. The amount of semen which leaves his body equals one or two teaspoons of fluid. The male has no control over the process, and seminal emissions may occur once in a while or, in some boys, several times a week. In this respect, too, each boy is different and the differences are normal.

You will discover that boys are disturbed at the idea of never knowing exactly when seminal emissions may occur, and they are embarrassed at the thought of soiling themselves or their bedding. Most boys seem immediately to assume that seminal emissions are like "wetting the bed." You will have to reassure them that although they cannot judge when this will happen (the way girls can usually predict the time of their menstrual periods), it is a natural function of the body and should be no cause for worry.

Boys are also concerned about the size of the penis and the difference between the circumcised and uncircumcised penis. (A frank discussion about the reasons for circumcision and the health routine necessary if a boy has not been circumcised should be discussed.) Emphasize that penis size varies greatly from male to male and that size has very little to do with a boy's "maleness" or his ability to become a father.

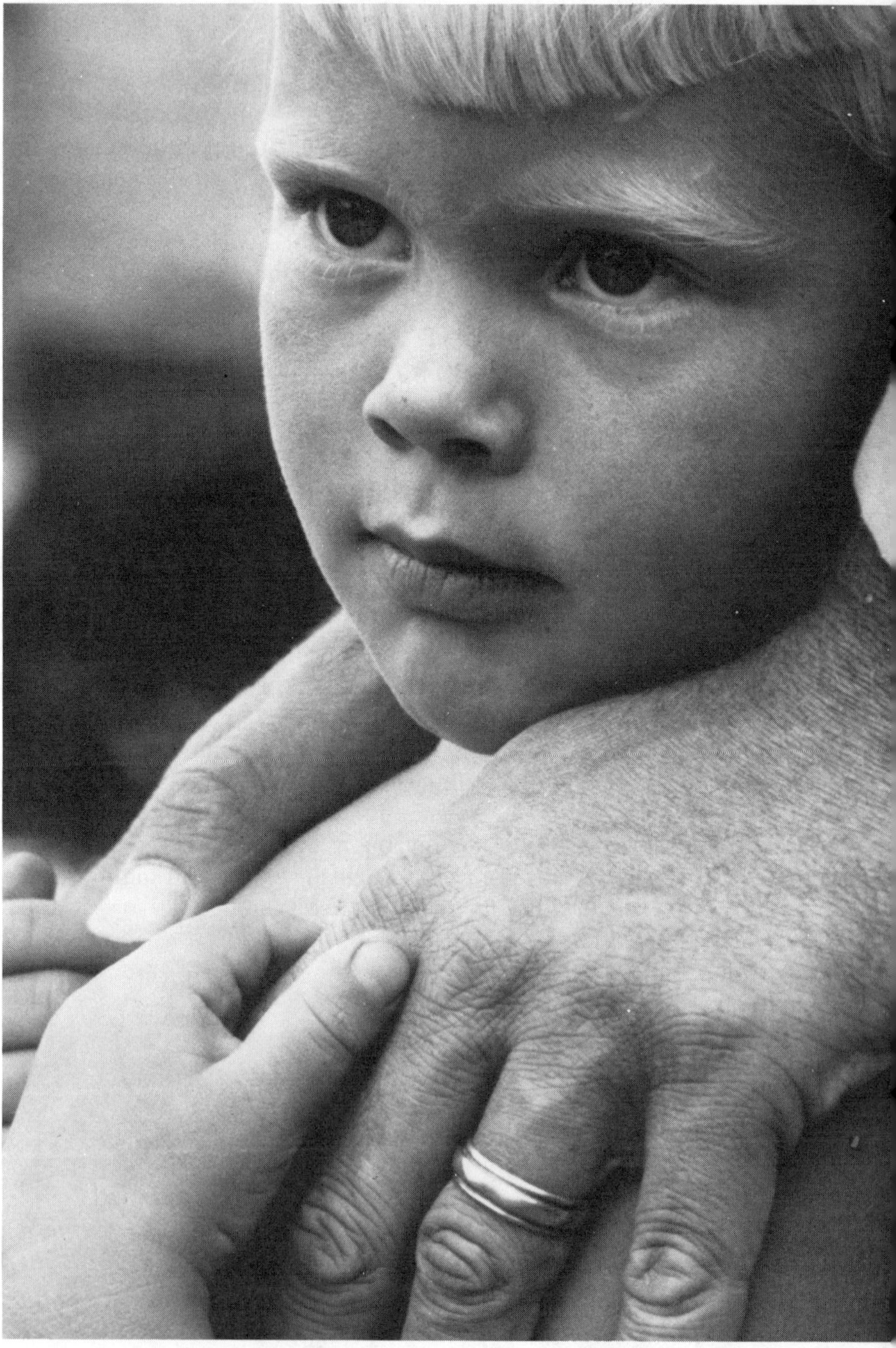

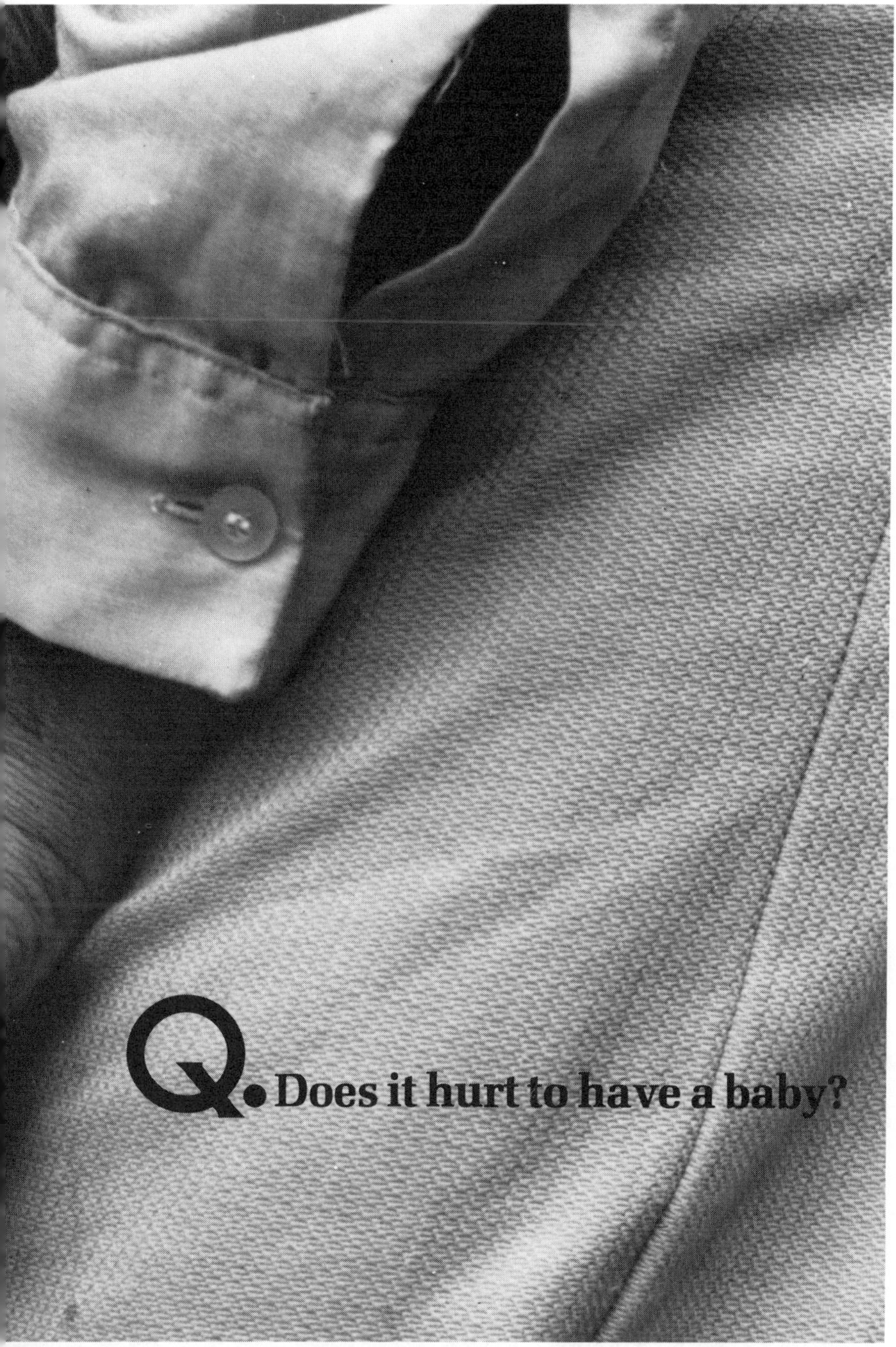

Q. Does it hurt to have a baby?

CHAPTER 8

QUESTIONS AND ANSWERS

DURING THE MANY years that we have been teaching sex education, we have learned that there is a definite pattern to the kinds of questions children ask at approximately each age level. Although there is overlapping and occasional questions way outside the normal pattern, kindergarten, first and second grade children are primarily interested in learning about how a baby develops inside its mother's body; third and fourth graders in how a baby is conceived and the sex act itself; intermediate grade children in the changes of puberty and the social and emotional aspects of sex.

The questions that follow are those that we have been asked most frequently, and are likely to come up in your group discussions. The questions are listed according to topic. The answers, stated in simplified form, are meant to serve as guidelines, and the questions are presented in an order which can carry your discussions forward. The topics become increasingly more sophisticated, but remember that some young children may ask questions you might normally expect from older children, and vice versa; it will be to your advantage to be familiar with all the topics. With some groups, you will feel it necessary to go into greater detail; with other groups less. As we indicated previously, when children want more information than you have given, they will ask for it. Start with a brief, simple answer and elaborate as the need arises.

PRENATAL DEVELOPMENT

Q: Where does a baby come from?

A: A baby comes from its mother's body. It grows in a special place called the uterus which keeps the baby warm and safe.

Q: Where is the uterus and what does it look like?

A: The uterus is located below the stomach. It is hollow and shaped something like a pear. It is about the size of a medium-sized pear, too.

Q: How does a baby eat and breathe before it is born?

A: Before it is born, a baby doesn't eat with its mouth or breathe through its nose the way we do. The unborn baby gets food and air from its mother's blood through a cord called the umbilical cord. One end of the cord is attached to the inside of the mother's uterus. The other end is attached to the baby's stomach.

Q: How does a baby go to the bathroom when it's inside its mother's body?

A: A baby's waste products leave its body through the umbilical cord and leave the mother's body when she goes to the bathroom.

Q: What happens to the cord after a baby is born?

A: After the baby is born, it no longer needs the umbilical cord to eat or breathe or eliminate, so the doctor cuts it and ties a small knot at the end to prevent it from bleeding. After about a week, the knot falls off and all that is left is the little round indentation that we call our bellybutton, or navel.

Q: Does it hurt the baby when the doctor cuts the cord?

A: No. There are no nerve endings in the cord, so cutting it feels just about the same as when you have your hair or your nails cut.

Q: How long does it take for a baby to grow in the uterus?

A: A baby is fully developed in about nine months.

Q: Can you tell whether a baby will be a girl or a boy before it's born?

A: Yes. There is a test that can be used, but it isn't done very often because it may harm the baby.

BIRTH

Q: How does a baby come out of its mother's body?

A: It comes out through a special opening between her legs called the vagina. The vagina is also called the birth canal. It is a passageway between the uterus and the outside of the woman's body.

Q: How can a baby come out of such a small place?

A: The vagina stretches and gets wide enough for the baby to come through.

Q: Which part of the baby comes out first?

A: Usually the head comes out first, stretching the vagina so that there is room enough for the body of the baby to follow. Sometimes a baby is born with its buttocks or feet first; this is called a breech birth.

Q: What happens to the vagina after the baby is born? Does it get small again?

A: After the baby is born, the vagina goes back to almost its original size.

Q: Does a baby come out of the same place where the mother goes to the bathroom?

A: No. The vagina is a separate opening behind the opening for liquid waste (urine), and in front of the opening for solid waste (feces). The opening for urine is called the urethra; the opening for solid waste is called the anus.

Q: Why do women go to the hospital to have their babies?

A: Not all women have their babies in a hospital, but most women do. Hospitals have doctors and nurses who can help the baby move from the inside to the outside of the mother's body.

Q: Does it hurt to have a baby?

A: It hurts some, but it need not be terribly painful. If necessary, a doctor can give the mother some pain-killing medicine.

Q: Why does the doctor slap the baby on the rear end after it's born?

A: The doctor slaps the baby to make it cry — this makes the baby's lungs expand, and the baby begins to breathe.

Q: How is a baby actually born?

A: When it is time for the baby to be born, the sides of the uterus begin to push and squeeze. The baby is usually ready and has its head downward. The uterus opens and the baby is pushed out through the vagina. Usually, a doctor helps to take the baby out.

Q: When a baby is first born, how can you tell whether it is a girl or a boy?

A: If it is a girl, it will have a vagina. If it is a boy, it will have a penis and testicles.

BREAST-FEEDING

Q: Do all mothers breast-feed their babies?

A: No. Some mothers don't have enough milk in their breasts; others prefer to feed their baby with bottled milk.

Q: How does the milk come out of the breast?

A: The milk is sucked out by the baby through openings in the mother's nipples.

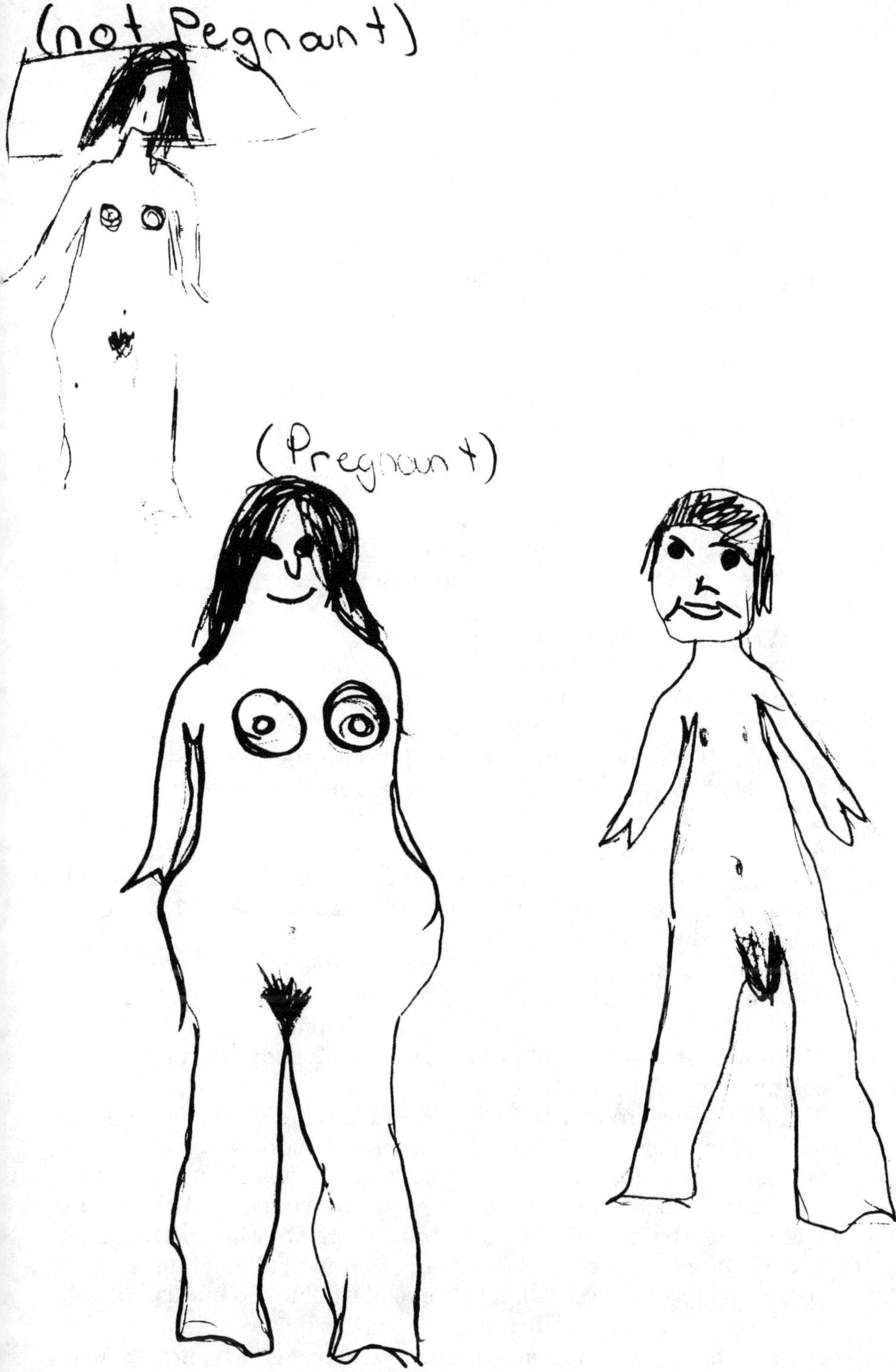
(not Pegnant)
(Pregnant)

Q: Do women always have milk in their breasts?
A: No. The only time they have milk in their breasts is right after the baby is born and as long as they continue to nurse.
Q: What happens to the milk if a mother doesn't nurse her baby?
A: The milk dries up. Usually, the doctor gives the woman some medicine to make the milk dry up faster.
Q: Does it hurt the mother when the baby breast-feeds?
A: No. In the early months, the baby has no teeth.

FERTILIZATION

Q: What makes a baby start to grow?
A: A baby starts to grow when a special cell inside the father's body, called a sperm cell, and a special cell inside the mother's body, called an egg cell, unite or join together.
Q: Where do sperm cells come from?
A: Sperm cells come from a part of the man's body called the testicles, or testes. The testicles are in a sac called the scrotum that hangs down behind the penis.
Q: Where do egg cells come from?
A: Egg cells come from two small parts of the woman's body called the ovaries. One ovary is on each side of the uterus.
Q: Do little boys have sperm cells?
A: No. A boy's body doesn't start to produce sperm cells until he is about 14 or 15 years old, or whenever he reaches puberty.
Q: Do little girls have egg cells?
A: Yes. When a girl baby is born, she already has more egg cells in her body than she will ever need; the egg cells have to mature or ripen, though, and this doesn't happen until she is about 11 or 12, or whenever she reaches puberty.
Q: Where do the egg cell and the sperm cell join together?
A: The egg cell and the sperm cell join inside the woman's body in a tube connected to the uterus called the Fallopian tube.
Q: How do sperm cells get inside the woman's body? How do the egg cell and the sperm cell get together?
A: Sperm cells are in a white liquid called semen, which comes out of the man's penis. The man puts his penis into the woman's vagina and puts the sperm cells there. This is called sexual intercourse or mating or making love. During sexual intercourse, the man puts millions of sperm cells in the woman's vagina. The sperm travel (swim) through the uterus and finally into the Fallopian tubes. If a sperm cell joins an egg cell, they travel back into the uterus.
Q: You mean a man really puts his penis inside a woman's body?
A: Yes, that's the way human beings are made. Our bodies are con-

structed so that a man and a woman fit together just right.

Q: Does it take only one egg and one sperm to begin a baby?

A: Yes. When a sperm cell enters and fertilizes the egg, the egg closes itself off so that no more sperm can enter.

Q: What happens to all the rest of the sperm?

A: The remaining sperm die and disintegrate after about three days.

Q: Why do some mothers have more than one baby at a time?

A: Once in a great while, a woman's ovaries discharge two eggs at a time instead of one; if the eggs are fertilized, the woman may have fraternal twins, or two children who don't look any more alike than most brothers and sisters. Even more rarely, a united egg and sperm may divide and develop into two or more identical parts, and the woman may have twins, triplets, etc. Since identical twins or triplets develop from the same egg and sperm, they are very much alike.

Q: If urine and semen both pass through the penis, how are they kept from mixing? In other words, can a man urinate into a woman's vagina while they are having sexual intercourse?

A: Urine and semen cannot come out of the penis at the same time. A valve automatically shuts off the urine when a man is having sexual intercourse.

Q: Do a husband and wife only have intercourse when they want to have a baby?

A: No. Most husbands and wives have intercourse many, many times, because it is a way for them to share their love for one another.

Q: If a man and a woman want to have sexual intercourse but they don't want to have a baby, what do they do?

A: They must prevent the sperm cells from reaching the egg cells. There are several different ways to do this and they are called birth control methods.

Q: Can a woman have a baby without being married?

A: Yes. A woman may be widowed or divorced after she conceives. Or she need not have been married when she first became pregnant.

Q: How can a woman tell if she is pregnant?

A: The most reliable sign of pregnancy is when a woman stops menstruating for a couple of months. A doctor can usually tell a woman soon after she misses a period whether or not she is pregnant.

Q: How old does a girl have to be before she can become pregnant?

A: A girl can become pregnant once she has gotten her first menstrual period.

Q: How old are most people when they start to have sexual relations?

A: This is up to the individual. Most people wait until they feel able to fully understand and cope with their emotions and actions.

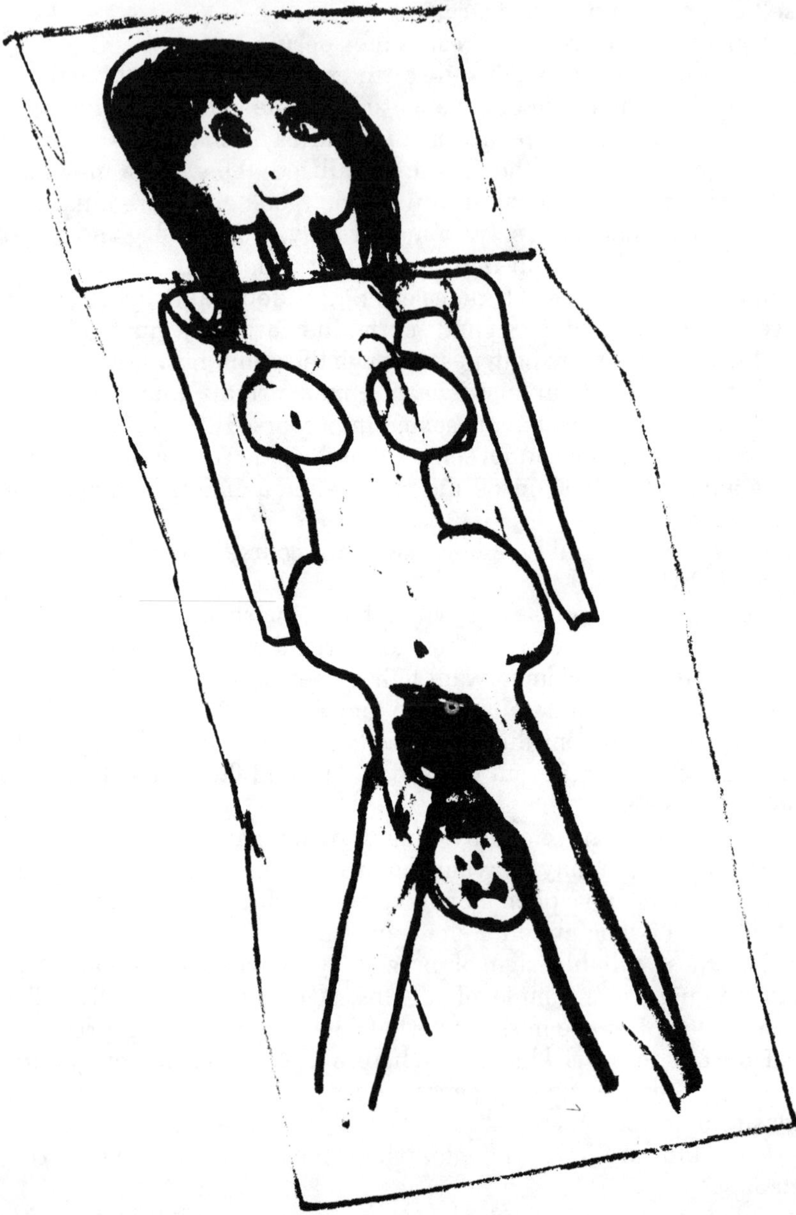

MENSTRUATION

Q: What is menstruation?

A: Every month a woman's uterus prepares to receive a fertilized egg. It does this by building up a lining of blood. If the woman's egg isn't fertilized, the lining of the uterus isn't needed and the body discharges it in the form of a bloody fluid. This process is called menstruation.

Q: At what age do girls usually start to menstruate?

A: Some girls begin to menstruate as early as 9 or 10, and some do not begin until they are 15 or 16. However, the average age is 12.

Q: How often does a girl menstruate and how long does the period usually last?

A: Most women have a menstrual period about every 28 days and the period can last anywhere from three days to a week. It should be kept in mind, however, that the number of days between periods and the number of days that a period lasts vary greatly from woman to woman. It should also be kept in mind that when a girl first starts to menstruate, her periods may be very irregular.

Q: Is it safe to take a bath when you are menstruating?

A: Yes. Bathing is not at all harmful while you are menstruating.

SEMINAL EMISSIONS

Q: What is a seminal emission, or "wet dream"?

A: When a boy reaches the age of 14 or 15, his sex glands begin to produce sperm cells; when a large supply builds up, some of these cells may pass out through the penis during sleep. The passage of semen is called a seminal emission, or nocturnal emission; it is also called a "wet dream" because it is frequently the result of a sexually exciting dream.

Q: Do all boys have seminal emissions?

A: Yes. Most boys begin to have "wet dreams" between the ages of 13 and 16.

Q: Can a boy become a father once he has begun to have "wet dreams"?

A: Yes, because this means that his body has begun to produce sperm cells.

MISCELLANEOUS QUESTIONS

Q: What is masturbation?

A: Masturbation is the rubbing of one's own genitals for pleasure and sexual excitement. Masturbation is perfectly normal and almost every boy and girl does it at one time or another.

Q: What is rape?

A: Rape is sexual intercourse forced upon an unconsenting person.

Q: What is circumcision?

A: Circumcision is the surgical removal of the foreskin, a loose piece of skin on the tip of the penis. Circumcision is usually performed a few days after birth for religious or personal hygiene reasons (it's easier to keep the penis clean if the foreskin is removed). Though not all boys are circumcised, doctors generally recommend it.

Q: What is a Caesarean birth?

A: A Caesarean birth is a surgical way to have a baby. Sometimes it isn't safe for a mother or her baby to deliver the child in the normal way, so the doctor makes a small cut in the uterus and lifts the baby out. Then he stitches the cut closed and it soon heals.

Q: What is an orgasm, or climax?

A: Orgasm, or climax, is the peak of sexual excitement. It is the final burst of pleasurable feeling which accompanies the release of muscular and nervous tension at the end of sexual intercourse. For both men and women, the sensation of orgasm is centered in the pelvic region; the penis and testicles in men, the clitoris, vagina and uterus in women. In the male, ejaculation or discharge of sperm accompanies orgasm. In the female, there is no comparable ejaculation. A woman does not have to experience orgasm in order to conceive. Orgasm can also result from masturbation or petting.

Q: What is an erection and what causes it?

A: An erection occurs when the penis becomes enlarged and rigid because its blood vessels are filled with an extra supply of blood. This condition is usually caused by sexual excitement, but it can also be caused by a full bladder or by almost any kind of excitement.

Q: What is an ejaculation?

A: An ejaculation is a discharge of semen from the penis. Semen is a milky fluid that contains millions of sperm cells. Ejaculation occurs when a man experiences orgasm.

Q: Does a man or a boy have an ejaculation every time he has an erection?

A: No, a man and especially a young boy or young man has many erections in which there is no ejaculation. There cannot, however, be an ejaculation without an erection.

Q: What is VD?

A: VD are initials which stand for venereal disease. Venereal diseases are infections contracted through sexual intercourse. The two most common types of VD in the United States are gonorrhea and syphilis.

Q: What is a contraceptive?

A: A contraceptive is a device or means of preventing a woman from becoming pregnant. Contraceptives are sometimes called birth control devices.

Q: What is incest?

A: Incest is having sexual intercourse with a close blood relative of the opposite sex. This is usually illegal, and dangerous for the child if the woman becomes pregnant.

Q: What is impotence?

A: Impotence is the inability to have an erection.

Q: What is a homosexual?

A: A homosexual is an adult who prefers having sexual relations with another adult of the same sex.

Q: What is a vasectomy?

A: A vasectomy is a minor operation which prevents sperm cells from leaving a man's body. In this operation, the tube which carries sperm cells from the testicles to the penis, the vas deferens, is severed and tied.

Q: What is necking?

A: Necking is generally thought of as light sex play, such as kissing and hugging.

Q: What is petting?

A: Petting is the caressing or fondling of the erotic, or sexual, parts of the body, primarily the breasts and the genitals. Petting is also called sexual foreplay because it helps to make the body ready for sexual intercourse.

The humanistic approach to sex education is a unique method whereby children acquire sexual information when they ask for it, by interacting with small groups of their peers and an adult discussion leader. We have given you the ideas and methods which have worked well in our groups and suggest that you adopt or adapt them to your situation. No matter what your environment or resources are, sex education should be a sharing process in which every child can gain a sense of his or her own worth and an appreciation for the feelings of others. The child who feels good about himself is receptive to absorbing knowledge. It is our belief that a positive self-image is the key to learning and understanding.

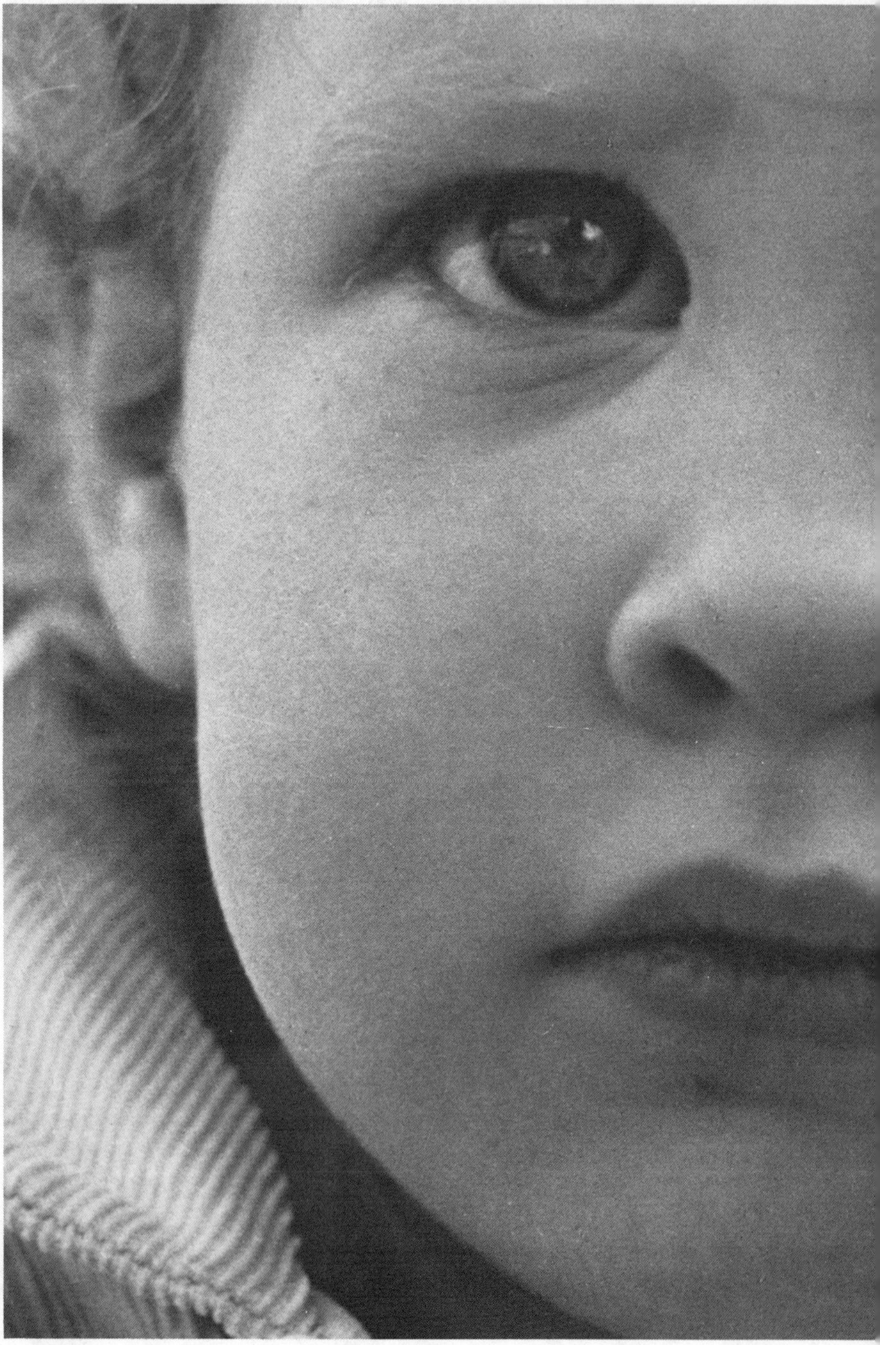

Q. How does a baby eat before it is born?

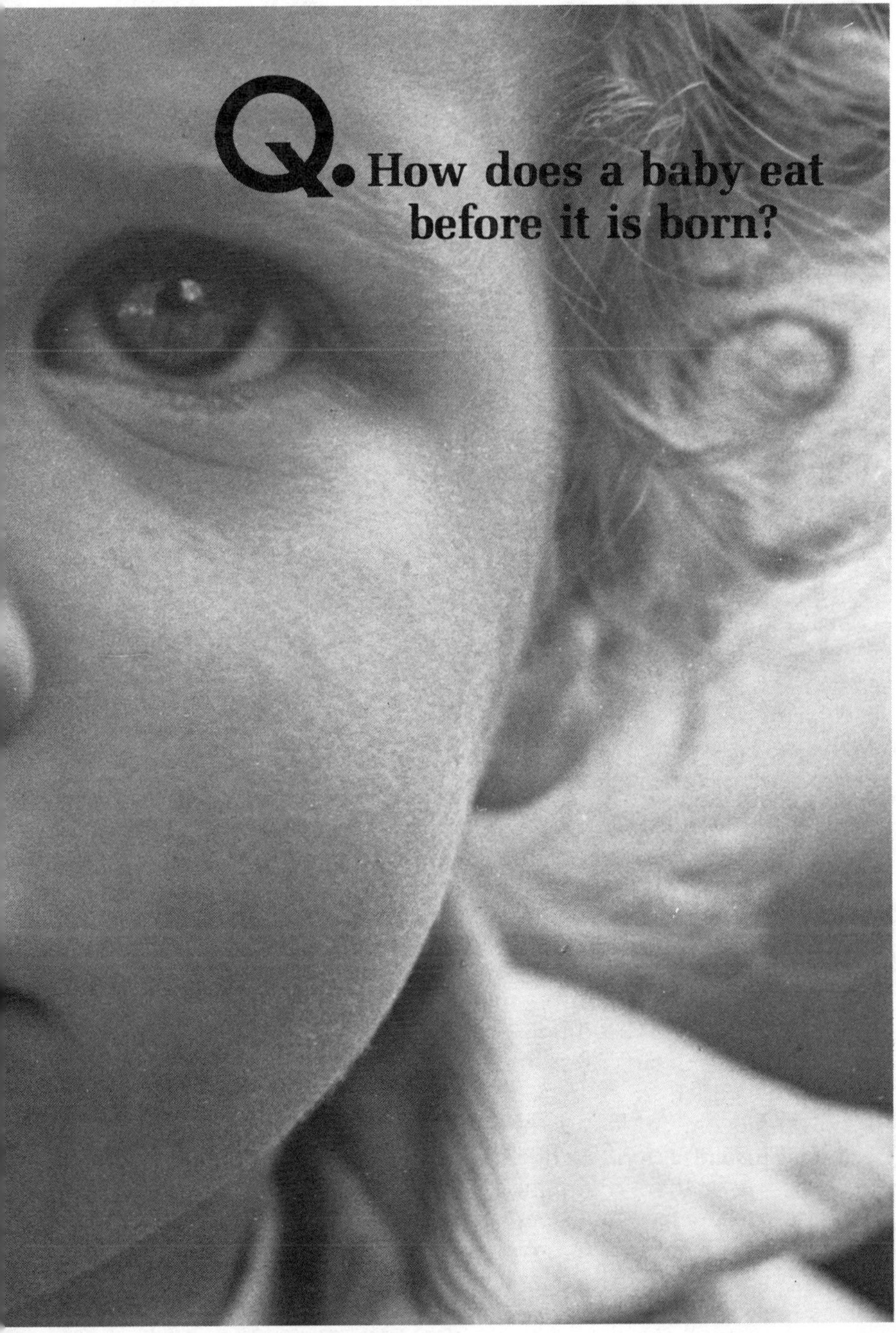

CHAPTER 9

GLOSSARY

Many of the following words probably will be discussed in your sex education groups. We have simplified their meanings so that you can easily explain them to children.

Abdomen — The part of the human body between the rib cage and the pelvis.

Abortion — The ending of a pregnancy; miscarriage. A natural, or spontaneous, abortion, takes place before the fourth month of pregnancy. The embryo comes loose from the wall of the uterus and is passed out of the mother's body through the birth canal. An abortion also may be performed as a medical treatment.

Acne — Pimples, blackheads and other skin eruptions that usually occur during adolescence; sometimes referred to as "adolescent skin."

Adolescence — The years during which the body of a child changes into that of an adult; the time of life between puberty and maturity.

Adoption — To take by choice into one's home a child born naturally to another, and to love and care for him as one's own.

Afterbirth — The placenta and other membranes that were used to nourish an unborn child in the womb. The afterbirth comes loose from the uterus and is expelled from the body through the birth canal shortly after the birth of the baby.

Amnion — The sac within the uterus that holds the unborn baby.

Amniotic Fluid — The fluid within the amnion that cushions and protects a baby during pregnancy.

Anus — The opening in the rectum through which solid waste (feces or bowel movement) leaves the body.

Artificial Insemination — The injection of sperm cells into the uterus by means other than sexual intercourse.

Athletic Supporter (Jockstrap)—protective device worn by men during athletic activity to cover the genitals.

Birth — The process through which a baby leaves the uterus and comes into the world.

Bladder — The sac within the body that holds urine.

Bowel Movement— The name given to the solid waste that leaves the body; also called feces.

Breast — Either of two milk-producing glands on a woman's chest; also called *bosom or bust.*

Breast-Feeding (Nursing) — Feeding a baby by having the infant suck milk from the breast.

Breech Birth — A form of birth in which a baby is born feet or buttocks first.

Buttocks (Butt) — The seat of the body, or the rump.

Caesarean Birth — A surgical way to deliver a baby if the mother cannot give birth through the birth canal. The doctor makes an incision in the abdominal wall and into the uterus and lifts the baby out. Then he stitches the incision and it soon heals.

Cell — The basic unit of life. Every living thing is made up of one or more cells.

Cervix — The narrow entrance into the uterus.

Chancre — A sore that is the first symptom of syphilis.

Chromosomes — The microscopic hairlike parts of the nucleus of a cell; they contain the genes that determine hereditary characteristics.

Circumcision — The surgical removal of the foreskin from the penis. Every male is born with a foreskin loosely covering the tip of the penis. It can be removed, by choice, for religious or personal hygiene reasons.

Clitoris — The small organ at the upper end of the female external genital area.

Conceive or Conception — To become pregnant; the fertilization of a female egg cell by a male sperm cell.

Congenital — Existing at birth; a result of heredity (usually referring to a disease).

Contraceptives — Devices used to prevent the fertilization of the egg

cell by the sperm cell.
Corpus Luteum(Yellow Body)— A mass of yellow tissue in the ovary formed after the ovarian follical (egg case) has released a mature egg. If the egg is fertilized, the corpus luteum releases a hormone that causes the lining of the uterus to thicken.
Divorce — The legal ending of a marriage.
Egg Cell — The reproductive cell of the female; the ovum.
Ejaculation — The discharge of semen from the penis which occurs at the climax of sexual excitement.
Embryo — The name given to the unborn baby within the uterus up until the tenth week after conception.
Endocrine Glands — Body parts that produce secretions that go to different parts of the body through the blood stream.
Endometrium — The lining of the uterus.
Erection — The penis in a rigid, hard state; the filling with blood of the tissues of the penis.
Estrogens — Female sex hormones, produced by the ovaries, which produce estrus, or sexual excitement, in women.
Fallopian Tubes(Uterine Tubes) — Two tubes, one on either side of the uterus, through which the egg cell travels from the ovary to the uterus. It is within one of these tubes that fertilization takes place.
Feces (Bowel Movement) — The solid waste matter formed in the bowel or intestine; it passes to the rectum and leaves the body through the anus in the process of defecation.
Female — Of the sex that is capable of bearing children; a woman or a girl.
Fertile — Able to produce children.
Fertilization — The union of an egg cell and a sperm cell.
Fetus — The term used to describe an unborn baby from the end of the third month of its development until birth. During the first ten weeks, the unborn baby is called an embryo.
Foreskin — The loose skin that fits over the tip of the penis.
Fraternal — Twins who developed from separately fertilized egg cells; identical twins developed from a single egg cell.
Genes — Tiny chemical substances found in the chromosomes of all cells; genes are the basic units of heredity.
Genitals — The external reproductive organs.
Germ Cell — Another name for a reproductive cell. A germ cell is either a male sperm or a female egg.
Gestation — The period of carrying a child in the uterus from fertilization to birth; pregnancy.
Gland — An organ which performs a specific bodily function.
Gonorrhea — A venereal disease which is transferred from person to

person by sexual contact.
Heredity — The process by which traits are passed from parents to offspring through genes in the reproductive cells.
Heterosexuality — The sexual attraction felt by members of one sex for members of the opposite sex.
Homosexuality — The sexual attraction felt by adults of one sex for adults of the same sex.
Hormones — Chemical substances which stimulate activity in the body. Produced in organs or endocrine glands, they are carried by the blood to other parts of the body where they help to regulate specific functions.
Hysterectomy — The surgical removal of the uterus.
Incest — Sexual relations between people closely related by blood, usually forbidden by law. The children born to close blood relatives are very likely to inherit any weakness present in the family.
Incubator — A container used to keep a premature or sick baby alive. It provides in a germ-proof environment the proper temperature and oxygen level that the baby needs. Egg incubators provide warmth for fertilized hen's eggs until they hatch.
Labia — The folds of skin in a female's vulva, or external genital area.
Labor — The term used to describe the uterine contractions during childbirth.
Lesbianism — Female homosexuality.
Litter — The term used in referring to the multiple offspring born at one time to animals.
Male — Of the sex that fertilizes egg cells; a man or a boy.
Mammal — A warm-blooded animal; female mammals give birth to live young and nurse their babies.
Masturbation — The act of touching or rubbing one's own genitals and getting sexual stimulation from the touch.
Mating—Joining in sexual intercourse. g.
Maturation — The process of growing and developing toward adulthood.
Menopause — The time in a woman's life when her ovaries stop releasing egg cells and her menstrual periods end, making her incapable of becoming pregnant. This usually happens when a woman is between 45 and 50 years old.
Menstruation — The monthly discharge of bloody fluid from the uterus through the vagina. This process begins at the onset of puberty and continues until the female reaches the menopause.
Miscarriage — The natural expulsion of an embryo or fetus from the uterus through the vagina; natural abortion. The fetus is usually less

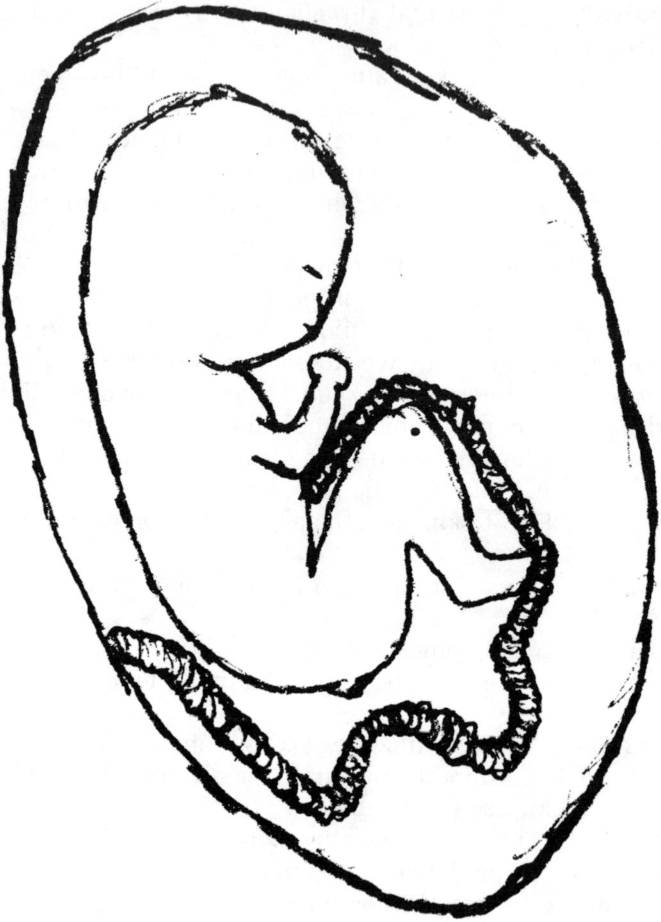

than 20 weeks old when a miscarriage occurs.

Multiple Birth — In humans, a multiple birth is the birth of two or more infants during the same time of labor; two infants are called twins, three are triplets, four are quadruplets, five are quintuplets, six are sextuplets and seven are septuplets.

Natural Childbirth — The birth of a baby in which the mother actively assists the delivery, rather than being asleep while it happens.

Navel — The small scar in the middle of the abdomen, usually called the bellybutton. It is the place where the umbilical cord was attached to a baby before its birth.

Obstetrician — A doctor who takes care of a woman during her pregnancy and childbirth.

Organ — A body part, or gland, composed of tissues.

Orgasm — The climax of sexual excitement. In the male, ejaculation of semen accompanies orgasm.

Ovaries — The female sex glands that produce egg cells.

Ovulation — The part of the female reproductive cycle during which a mature egg is released from one of the ovaries.

Ovum — The female reproductive cell.

Pelvis — The bony structure in the lower part of the abdomen that shelters the inner reproductive organs.

Penis — The tubelike male sex organ.

Period — A term used to describe the time of the month when a female has a menstrual discharge.

Pituitary Gland — The gland, or body part, that controls body growth.

Placenta — The mass of blood vessels and tissues attached to the wall of the uterus during pregnancy; it enables a developing baby to get oxygen and nourishment from its mother, and to eliminate waste matter.

Pregnancy — The condition of a female who has a developing baby in her uterus.

Premature Birth — A birth is considered premature when a baby is born two or more weeks earlier than the normal gestation period of nine months. A premature baby usually weighs less than five pounds.

Prostitute — A woman who has sexual relations for money.

Puberty — The years during which youngsters begin to mature sexually and become adults; the time when it is first possible to fertilize egg cells or bear children. The onset of puberty varies from individual to individual, girls usually maturing around twelve, about two years earlier than boys.

Pubic Hair — The hair that grows in both the female and male external genital areas; the development of pubic hair is one of the first signs of the approach of puberty.

Rape — Sexual intercourse forced on an unconsenting person.

Rectum — The end of the large intestine where solid bodily waste accumulates. The waste then leaves the body through the anus.

Reproduction — The process through which animals bring a new life into the world.

Reproductive Organs — The sex organs which make reproduction possible.

Scrotum — The sac of skin in male mammals which hangs under the penis outside of the body and contains the testicles.

Secondary Sex Characteristics — The physical features other than the external sex organs which cause the male and the female to differ in outward appearance.

Semen — The thick whitish fluid containing sperm cells which is ejaculated from the penis during orgasm.

Seminal Emission — An ejaculation of semen which usually takes place at night; nocturnal emission or "wet dream."

Sex — Either of two organisms called male and female. Also, the inborn instinct that causes males and females to be attracted to each other and have sexual intercourse.

Sex Hormones — Chemical substances in the body which control all sexual characteristics of an individual.

Sexual Intercourse — The physical union of a man and a woman during which the penis enters the vagina. Also called "making love," coitus and copulation.

Siamese Twins — Identical twins who are joined at one part of their bodies.

Sperm — The male reproductive cell.

Sterility — The inability to reproduce.

Sterilization — The process of making an individual incapable of reproducing.

Stillbirth — The birth of a dead baby after at least 28 weeks of pregnancy.

Syphilis — A venereal disease spread by sexual contact.

Tampon — A tube of absorbent material inserted into the vagina to absorb the monthly menstrual discharge.

Testicles (Testes) — The male reproductive glands which produce sperm. The testicles are located in a sac called the scrotum, which is directly below the base of the penis.

Twins — Two babies carried in the uterus at the same time and born within a short time of one another. Twins can result from two egg cells meeting with two sperm cells (fraternal) or one egg cell meeting with one sperm cell and dividing in half to form two babies (identical).

Umbilical Cord — A ropelike structure which connects a developing baby (at its abdomen) to the placenta; through this tube the baby receives nourishment and oxygen and eliminates waste.
Umbilicus — The navel, or bellybutton.
Urethra — A tube from the bladder through which urine leaves the body. In the female, the outside opening of the urethra is in the vulva in front of the vaginal opening. In the male, the urethra also acts as a tube for semen but never carries both semen and urine at the same time.
Urine — The yellowish liquid waste matter which leaves the body through the urethra. Formed in the kidneys, urine passes to the bladder, accumulates there and then leaves the body through the process of urination.
Uterus — The pear-shaped reproductive organ in the lower part of the female body where a baby grows and is nourished until birth.
Vagina — A tube inside the opening between a female's legs which leads to the uterus. A baby passes along the vagina to the outside world during childbirth. The vagina is also called the birth canal.
Vas Deferens — The tube that carries sperm from the testicles to the urethra.
Venereal Disease (VD) — Any of several diseases, usually contracted through sexual intercourse. Two of the most common types of venereal disease in this country are gonorrhea and syphilis.
Virginity — The state of being a virgin, or a male or female who has never had sexual intercourse.
Vulva — The external genital area of the female which includes the opening to the vagina.
Womb — Another name for the uterus.

Q. Does it hurt the baby when the doctor cuts the cord?

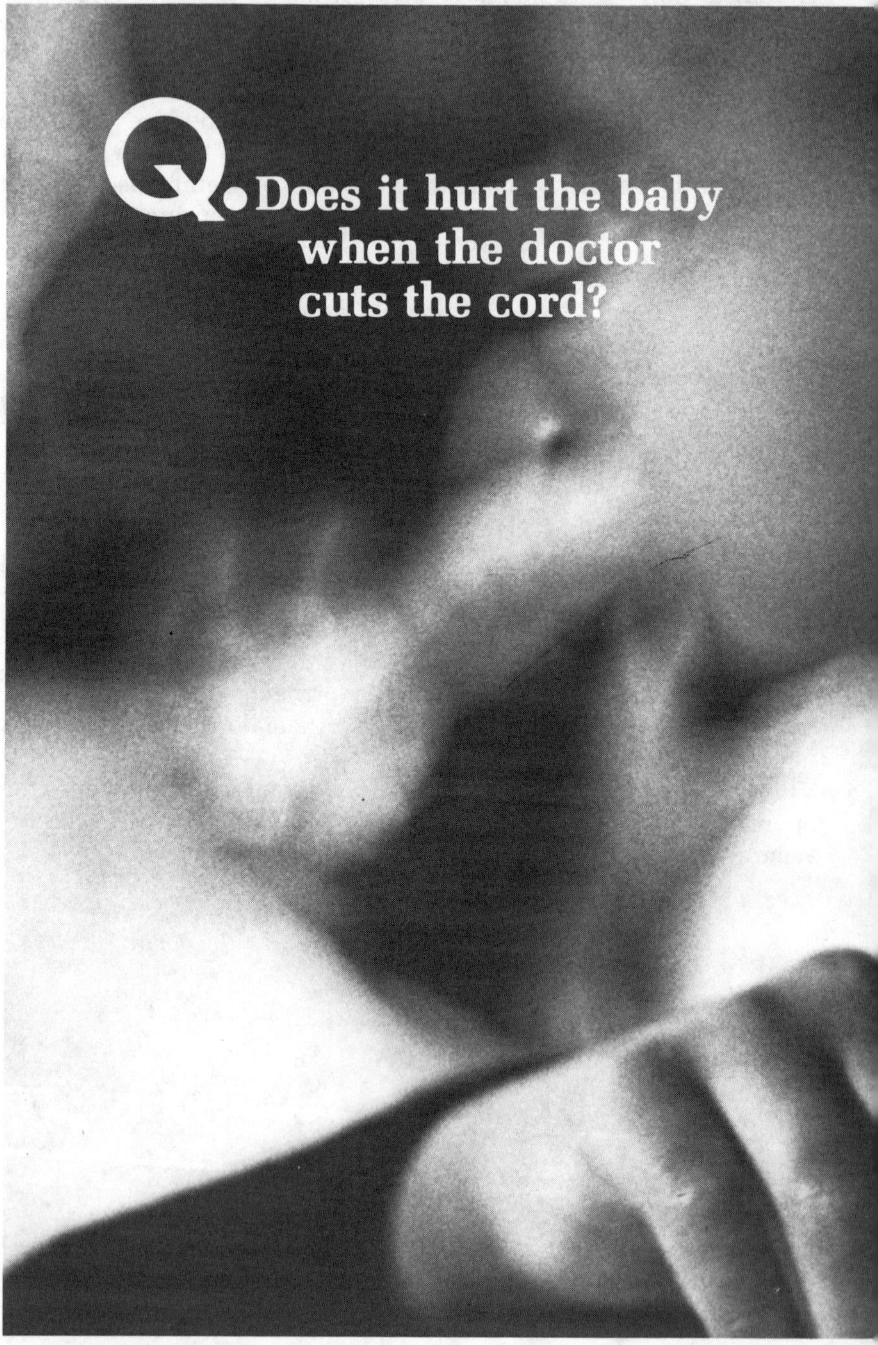

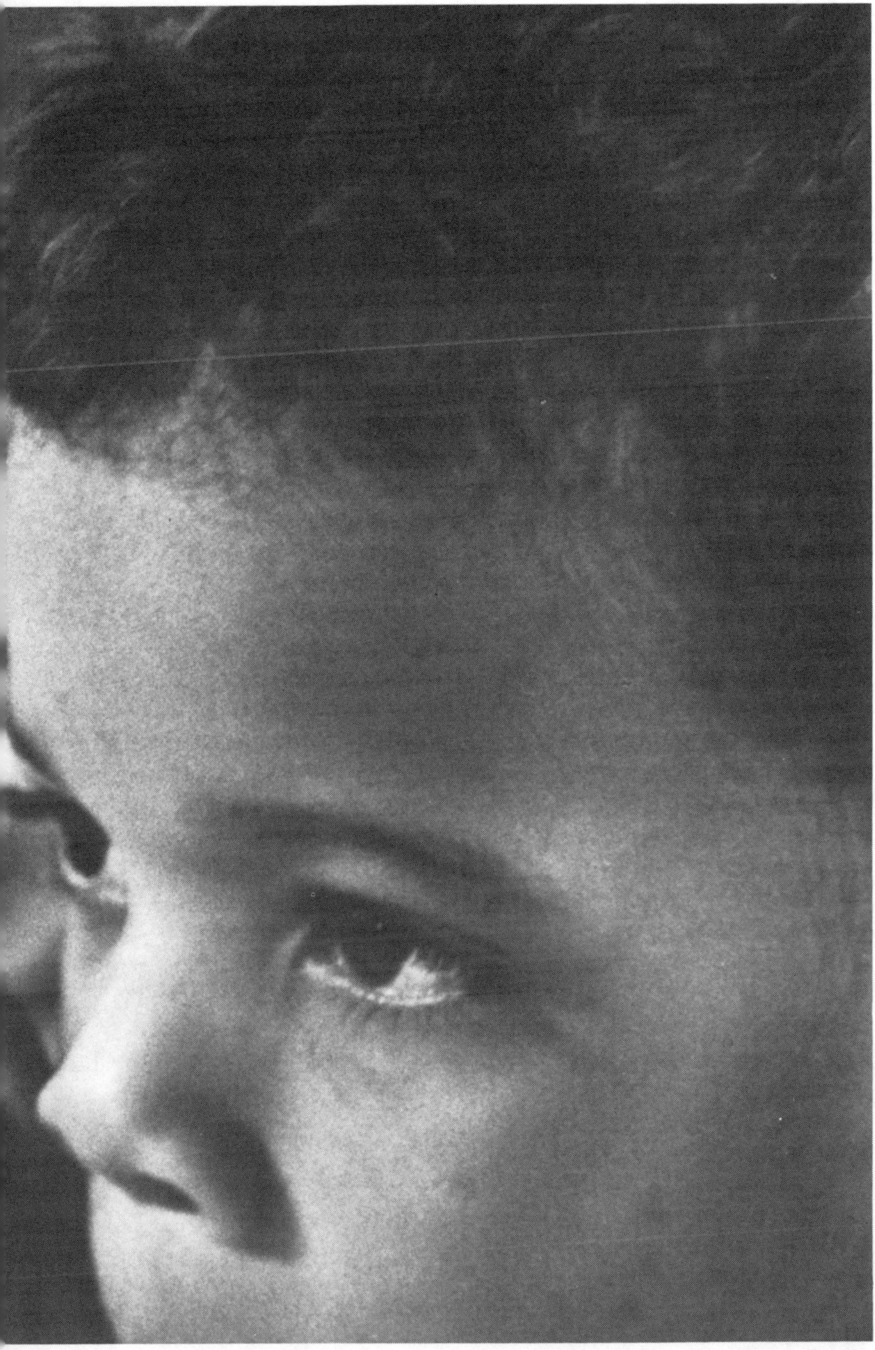

CHAPTER 10

RESOURCES

We have found the following materials and sources to be very helpful in teaching sex education.

WRITTEN FOR ADULTS

Arnstein, Helene S. *Your Growing Child And Sex*. New York: Avon, 1968.

Berne, Eric. *What Do You Say After You Say Hello?* New York: Grove Press, 1972.

Child Study Association of America. *What To Tell Your Child About Sex*. New York: Child Study Press, 1974.

Child Study Association of America. *When Children Ask About Sex*. New York: Child Study Press, 1974 (rev. ed.).

Uslander, Arlene et al. *Their Universe: The Study Of A Unique Sex Education Program For Kids*. New York: Delacorte, 1973.

WRITTEN FOR GRADES K — 3

Gruenberg, Sidonie, and Gruenberg, Benjamin. *The Wonderful Story of You*. New York: Doubleday, 1960.

Hobson, Laura Z. *I'm Going To Have A Baby*. New York: John Day Co., 1967.

Levine, Milton, and Seligmann, Jean. *A Baby Is Born*. New York: Golden Press, 1966 (out of print).

Selsam, Millicent. *All About Eggs*. Reading, Ma.: Addison-Wesley, 1952.

Strain, Frances Bruce. *Being Born*. New York: Hawthorn Books, 1970 (rev. ed.).

WRITTEN FOR GRADES 4 — 5

Andry, Andrew C., and Schepp, Steven. *How Babies Are Made*. New York: Time-Life, 1968.

Dalton, Katherine. *The Menstrual Cycle*. New York: Pantheon, 1971.

Hofstein, S., and Richmond J. *The Human Story — Facts On Birth, Growth, And Reproduction*. Glenview, Il.: Scott Foresman & Co., 1972.

Le Shan, Eda. *What Makes Me Feel This Way*. New York: Macmillan, 1972.

Protal, Colette. *The Beauty Of Birth*. New York: Alfred A. Knopf, 1971.

Showers, Paul. *Baby Starts To Grow*. New York: Crowell Co., 1969.

Shultz, Gladys D. *It's Time You Knew*. Philadelphia: J.B. Lippincott, 1955.

WRITTEN FOR GRADES 6 — 8

Duvall, Evelyn. *Love And The Facts of Life*. New York: Association Press, 1967.

Gordon, Sol. *Facts About Sex: A Basic Guide*. New York: John Day Co., 1973.

Johnson, Eric. *Love And Sex In Plain Language*. Philadelphia: J.B. Lippincott, 1974.

Pomeroy, Wardell. *Boys And Sex*. New York: Delacorte, 1968.

Pomeroy, Wardell. *Girls And Sex*. New York: Delacorte, 1969.

BOOKLETS

Bernhagen, Lillian F. *What A Miracle You Are Boys.* Indianapolis: Bobbs-Merrill, 1968.

Lerrigo, Marion O., and Cassidy, Michael. *A Doctor Talks To Nine To Twelve Year Olds.* Chicago: Budlong Press, 1969.

Levine, Milton I., and Seligmann, Jean H. *Human Reproduction.* New York: Harper & Row, 1967 (out of print).

Meilach, Dona Z., and Mandel, Elias, *A Doctor Talks To Five To Eight Year Olds.* Chicago: Budlong Press, 1969.

VENEREAL DISEASE INFORMATION

Grover, John W., and Grace, Dick. *VD: The ABC's.* Englewood Cliffs, N.J.: Prentice-Hall, 1971.

Some Questions and Answers About VD. American Social Health Association, 1740 Broadway, New York, NY 10019.

Syphilis And Gonorrhea. Institute for Sex Education, 162 N. State St., Chicago, IL 60601.

Teacher's Handbook On Venereal Disease Education. William F. Schwartz, American Association of Health, Physical Education and Recreation, 1201 16th St., N.W., Washington, D.C. 20036.

PLEASE RETURN TO LIBRARY
PLANNED PARENTHOOD: SHASTA-DIABLO
2185 PACHECO STREET
CONCORD, CA 94520
(510) 676-0505